MCQs IN BASIC SCIENCE OPHTHALMOLOGY

MCQs IN BASIC SCIENCE OPHTHALMOLOGY

JOHN FERRIS, FRCOphth
The Western Ophthalmic Hospital, London

BMJ
Publishing
Group

To my parents

First published in 1994
by the BMJ Publishing Group, BMA House, Tavistock Square,
London WC1H 9JR

British Library Cataloguing in Publication Data

A catalogue record for this book is available
from the British Library

ISBN 0–7279–0795–6

Typeset, printed and bound in Great Britain by
Latimer Trend & Company Ltd., Estover, Plymouth

Contents

Foreword		ix
Preface		xi
Acknowledgements		xiii

Ocular anatomy   **1**

1	The orbit and paranasal sinuses	1
2	The lacrimal system	5
3	The eyelids	9
4	The conjunctiva	14
5	The cornea	16
6	The ciliary body	22
7	The iris	24
8	The lens	29
9	The choroid and sclera	31
10	The retina	35
11	Anterior visual pathways	42
12	The extraocular muscles	48
13	The cranial nerves	52
14	Autonomic nervous system of the head and neck	58
15	Orbital blood vessels and cavernous sinus	64
16	Skull osteology	69
17	Gross anatomy of the head and neck	74
	Answers	84

Microbiology   **86**

1	General microbiology	86
2	Cocci	91
3	Bacilli	93
4	Chlamydia	100
5	General virology	101
6	Herpes viruses	105
7	Airborne and enteric viruses	109
8	Hepatitis B and HIV	112
9	Fungi	118
10	Protozoa	120
11	Antimicrobial agents	125
	Answers	133

Pathology **135**
1 Inflammation 135
2 Immunology 146
3 Hypersensitivity reactions 154
4 Transplantation immunology 159
5 Cardiovascular pathology: thrombosis 162
6 Cardiovascular pathology: atherosclerosis 166
7 Neoplasia 169
Answers 177

Pharmacology **178**
1 Pharmacokinetics 178
2 Cholinergic agonists 180
3 The adrenergic system 184
4 Hyperosmotic agents and carbonic anhydrase
  inhibitors 187
5 Corticosteroids 189
6 Ocular anaesthetics 192
7 Antimitotic and immunosuppressive
  chemotherapy 193
8 Ocular side effects of systemic
  medications 194
Answers 195

Ocular physiology **196**
1 The lacrimal apparatus 196
2 The eyelids 199
3 The cornea 202
4 The aqueous and intraocular pressure PA Bloom 207
5 The lens 216
6 Accommodation 220
7 The vitreous 224
8 The pupil 228
9 The extraocular muscles and ocular
  movements 239
10 The retina 248
11 Electrodiagnostic tests 261
12 The visual pathways 272
13 Visual acuity and adaptation GB Arden 277
14 Colour vision GB Arden 290
15 Binocular vision and stereopsis 292
Answers 297

General physiology   **299**
  1 Cardiovascular physiology   299
  2 Respiratory physiology   305
  3 Endocrinology   309
  4 Renal physiology   317
  5 Muscle physiology   325
  6 The central nervous system   331
  Answers   334

Index   335

Foreword

Multiple choice questions remain a favoured method of examination, and so practice using the technique is essential. Although essay questions and viva voce are essential components of some examinations, the first part of the Fellowship of the Royal College of Ophthalmology uses MCQs as its method of choice. The advantages are considerable: there can be a wide coverage in a short period of time, the marking is objective, feedback is precise, and computers can be used in marking. The disadvantage is that the questions are often difficult to set.

In spite of the objectivity of the method, it is known that skill and strategy are an important component in determining success or failure: hence the need for a manual that illustrates the kind of questions that may appear. For those in particular who have not been exposed to the method, the series of probing questions will be both informative and practical in understanding and practising the techniques that are employed in construction of MCQs.

This text will serve to refresh people's memories, and to pinpoint areas of individual weakness. It reviews most of the areas that are covered in Part I of the FRCOphth examination. John Ferris has collected an impressive array of questions that will serve as a useful revision of the basic sciences, particularly as applied to ophthalmology. It cannot be regarded as a short cut to the process of learning from texts, lectures and practical experience, but it will surely indicate to candidates whether the time is ripe to sit the examination.

David Easty
Professor of Ophthalmology,
University of Bristol 1994

Preface

For all ophthalmologists in training the first academic hurdle to be negotiated is the primary fellowship examination. This examination expects candidates to have not only a detailed knowledge of ocular physiology, anatomy, and pharmacology, but also a sound grounding in general physiology, pathology, and head and neck anatomy. These later topics are ones that candidates frequently neglect, to their cost! This book is aimed primarily at candidates about to sit the primary fellowship examination, and at final fellowship candidates who may need to reacquaint themselves with the ocular basic sciences. The 500 or so multiple choice questions which comprehensively cover all the topics detailed above will, I hope, provide not only practice for the exam but also a useful means of self-assessment with which candidates can critically monitor their revision.

However, this book was never intended to be solely a "practice" MCQ text and it differs from other books of this ilk in a number of key areas. The questions have been structured so that explanations for the answers given can be incorporated into summary paragraphs. Additional information, not directly related to the preceding question, has also been incorporated into these paragraphs, which are often accompanied by simple diagrams or illustrations. They thus form a concise synopsis of the topic covered in each chapter, which may be read independently of the preceding questions enabling the book to be used as a revision text (in conjunction with recommended reference texts). It is hoped that the structured nature of these paragraphs will also be helpful when planning short note answers and essays, both of which form an integral part of the fellowship examinations.

Success in postgraduate examinations requires a modicum of good luck; however, there is no substitute for meticulous preparation and practice of examination techniques. The "secret" of success is summed up in the barbed retort of the golfer Gary Player, after a journalist unwisely suggested that he had been lucky to win a tournament: "It's funny, but the more I practise, the luckier I become!" It is hoped that this book will make the practice a little less arduous, and ultimately rewarding.

Acknowledgements

The help of the following people in reviewing sections of the text is gratefully acknowledged:

GB Arden (Visual acuity and adaptation, Temporal responsiveness of vision, Colour vision)
Alan C Bird (Retina)
RJC Cooling (Vitreous)
Linda Ficker (Cornea)
D Flitcroft and JF Acheson (Visual pathways)
GE Holder (Electrodiagnostic tests)
JP Lee (Extraocular muscles and ocular movements, Binocular vision and stereopsis)
BR Mackenna (Physiology)
Alison CE McCartney (Pathology)
MH Miller (Aqueous and intraocular pressure)
Carlos Pavesio (Pharmacology, Microbiology)
Geoffrey Rose (Lacrimal apparatus and eyelids)
MD Sanders (Pupil)
RAW Weale (Accommodation)
Bernard Wood (Anatomy)

Special thanks are also due to Ann Young and Sue Tedd for their patience in typing the manuscript.

Ocular anatomy

1: The orbit and paranasal sinuses

1.1 *Orbit*

a. The lateral wall is formed by the frontal and zygomatic bones
b. The palatine bone lies in the medial wall
c. The superior orbital fissure is in the lesser wing of the sphenoid bone
d. Whitnall's tubercle is found on the zygomatic bone
e. The roof is made solely from the frontal bone

The bony orbit is a pear-shaped cavity that is made from constituents of seven individual bones. The thin orbital floor is formed primarily by the orbital plate of the maxilla with contributions from the zygomatic and palatine bones. The lateral wall is formed by the zygomatic bone (on which lies Whitnall's tubercle) and the greater wing of the sphenoid posteriorly. The orbital roof is formed predominantly by the orbital plate of the frontal bone with contributions from the lesser wing of the sphenoid bone. The maxilla, lacrimal, ethmoid and body of the sphenoid all contribute to the thin medial wall of the orbit. The superior orbital fissure at the orbital apex lies between the greater and lesser wings of the sphenoid bone.

1.2 *Relations and connections of the orbit*

The orbit:
a. Is separated from the ethmoidal air cells by the lamina papyrecia
b. Is connected to the pterygopalatine fossa by the inferior orbital foramen
c. Is in communication with the middle cranial fossa via the superior orbital fissure
d. Lies superior to the maxillary sinus
e. Is connected to the middle meatus via the nasolacrimal duct

The orbit has a number of important relations with the paranasal sinuses. It is separated from the ethmoidal air cells by the
lamina papyrecia, and ethmoidal mucoceles may break through
this thin barrier causing proptosis of the globe. Fractures of the
orbital floor may result in herniation of orbital contents into the
maxillary sinus, e.g. blowout fractures. The orbit is connected
to the pterygopalatine fossa via the inferior orbital fissure and to
the middle cranial fossa via the superior orbital fissure. The
nasolacrimal duct connects the orbit to the inferior meatus of
the nose.

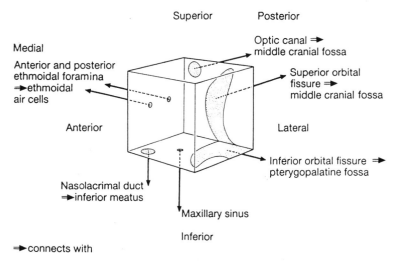

Fig 1 Schematic diagram of the relations and connections of the left orbit

1.3 *Contents of the orbital fissures and canals*

a. The optic nerve, ophthalmic artery and vein are all found
   in the optic canal
b. The lacrimal nerve passes through the superior orbital
   fissure outside the tendinous ring
c. The abducent nerve passes through the superior orbital
   fissure outside the tendinous ring
d. The inferior orbital fissure transmits branches of the
   maxillary nerve
e. The oculomotor nerve divides after passing through the
   superior orbital fissure

The optic canal contains the optic (with its meningeal coverings) and the ophthalmic artery, the ophthalmic vein being found in the superior orbital fissure. The lacrimal, frontal and trochlear nerves pass through the superior orbital fissure above the tendinous ring, whereas the nasociliary, abducent and both divisions of the oculomotor nerve pass though the superior orbital fissure inside the tendinous ring. The inferior orbital fissure is continuous with the infraorbital canal and transmits branches of the maxillary nerve, plus an emissary vein connecting the ophthalmic vein to the pterygoid plexus.

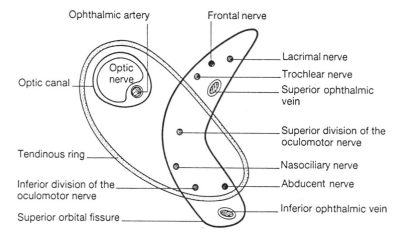

Fig 2 Contents of the superior orbital fissure and optic canal

1.4 *Paranasal sinuses*

a. All air sinuses, except the ethmoidal sinuses, are normally present at birth
b. Sinuses are lined by a stratified squamous epithelium
c. The maxillary sinus drains via the hiatus semilunaris
d. The sphenoidal sinus drains into the superior meatus of the nose
e. Ethmoidal sinuses drain into the middle and superior meatuses of the nose

All paranasal sinuses are normally present at birth (apart from the frontal sinus which is rudimentary until 2 years of age). All sinuses are lined by a pseudostratified columnar ciliated epithelium, which aids the passage of mucus into the nasal cavity. The maxillary sinus drains via the hiatus semilunaris into the middle meatus of the nose. The anterior and middle ethmoidal air cells, along with the frontal air cells, also drain into the middle meatus of the nose. The posterior ethmoidal air cells drain into the superior meatus whereas the sphenoidal air drain into the sphenoethmoidal recess.

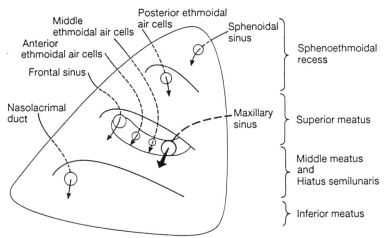

Fig 3 Schematic diagram of paranasal sinus drainage (lateral wall of the right nasal cavity)

1.5 *Innervation and lymphatic drainage of the paranasal sinuses*

a. The ophthalmic division of the trigeminal innervates the frontal sinuses
b. Branches of the nasociliary nerve provide the majority of the innervation to the ethmoidal sinuses
c. The maxillary sinus is innervated by the infraorbital, anterior, middle and posterior superior alveolar nerves
d. Lymph from the maxillary sinus drains to retropharyngeal nodes
e. Lymph from the frontal sinus drains to submandibular nodes

A knowledge of the paranasal sinuses innervation explains the distribution of referred pain from sinus infection. The frontal sinus is innervated by the supraorbital nerve (a branch of the ophthalmic division of the trigeminal), which also supplies the skin of the forehead and scalp, so explaining the distribution of referred pain in patients with frontal sinusitis. Likewise, maxillary sinusitis may cause referred pain in the upper teeth and the skin of the cheek because of their innervation by the infraorbital, anterior, middle, and posterior superior alveolar nerves. The ethmoidal sinuses are supplied by the anterior and posterior ethmoidal nerves, and by branches of the pterygopalatine ganglion. All lymph drainage from the paranasal sinuses is to the submandibular nodes, except the sphenoidal sinuses and posterior ethmoidal sinuses which drain into the retropharyngeal group of nodes.

2: The lacrimal system

2.1 Lacrimal gland structure

a. The lacrimal gland consists of two equally sized lobes
b. The lacrimal gland lies within a definite capsule
c. The lacrimal ducts open into the superior fornix via the palpebral lobe
d. The gland lies wholly behind the orbital system
e. The two lobes of the gland are separated by the levator muscle

The lacrimal gland is a bilobed gland, possessing no definitive capsule, which lies superotemporally in the orbit behind the orbital septum. The orbital lobe is the larger of the two and is continuous with the smaller palpebral lobe around the lateral border of the levator palpebrae aponeurosis. The palpebral lobe lies below the aponeurosis and extends into the upper eyelid. Lacrimal ducts arising in the orbital lobe pass through the palpebral lobe and into the superior fornix of the conjunctiva, along with additional ducts that arise from the palpebral part of the gland.

2.2 *Parasympathetic innervation of the lacrimal gland*

a. Preganglionic secretomotor fibres arise in the superior salivatory nucleus
b. Preganglionic fibres travel in the nervus intermedius
c. Preganglionic fibres approach the pterygoid canal in the lesser petrosal nerve
d. Preganglionic fibres synapse in the ciliary ganglion
e. Preganglionic fibres "hitchhike" to the gland on branches of the maxillary and ophthalmic nerves

The parasympathetic supply to the lacrimal gland arises in the superior salivatory nucleus, one of the nuclei of the parasympathetic brain stem. Fibres travelling in the nervus intermedius leave the middle ear as the greater petrosal nerve, which enters the middle cranial fossa. The greater petrosal and deep petrosal nerves combine in the pterygoid canal, which opens into the pterygopalatine fossa. The preganglionic fibres synapse in the pterygopalatine ganglion, and postganglionic fibres "hitchhike" along the infraorbital, zygomaticotemporal and lacrimal nerves to the lacrimal gland.

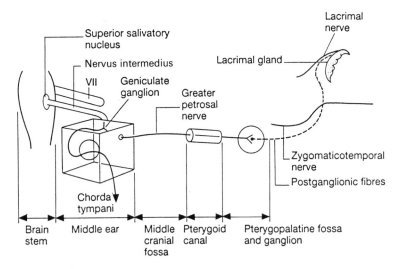

Fig 4 Innervation of the lacrimal gland

2.3 Lacrimal gland histology

a. The lacrimal gland is a lobulated tubuloacinar structure
b. Acinar cells have an apically located nucleus
c. Acinar cells are rich in rough endoplasmic reticulum, golgi apparatus and mitochondria
d. Large ducts are surrounded by myoepithelial cells
e. Large ducts have a single layered epithelium

The lacrimal gland is a lobulated tubuloacinar gland. Acinar cells, which have a predominantly serous secretion, are characterised by their basally located nuclei and are rich in rough endoplasmic reticulum, golgi apparatus, and mitochondria. A basement membrane separates these cells from the surrounding myoepithelial cells. The larger intralobular ducts have a two layered epithelial lining whereas smaller ducts are lined only by a single layer of cuboidal cells. Both are ringed by myoepithelial cells, which have contractile properties.

2.4 Lacrimal drainage

a. Lacrimal canaliculi run horizontally throughout their length and measure 10 mm
b. The common canaliculus pierces the lacrimal sac 2.5 mm below its apex
c. The common canaliculus lies in front of the medial palpebral ligament
d. The lacrimal canaliculi may enter the sac separately
e. The lacrimal canaliculi are surrounded by fibres of the orbicularis oculi

A knowledge of lacrimal canaliculus anatomy is important when conducting lacrimal probing. The canaliculi are L shaped structures with a short (2 mm) vertical portion and a longer (10 mm) horizontal portion. They normally unite to form a common canaliculus, which lies behind the medial palpebral ligament and pierces the lacrimal sac 2.5 mm below its apex. On occasions the canaliculi may enter the sac separately. The lacrimal canaliculi are surrounded by fibres continuous with the lacrimal component of the orbicularis oculi, which by its contraction aids the pumping action of tears from the lacrimal canaliculi into the lacrimal sac.

7

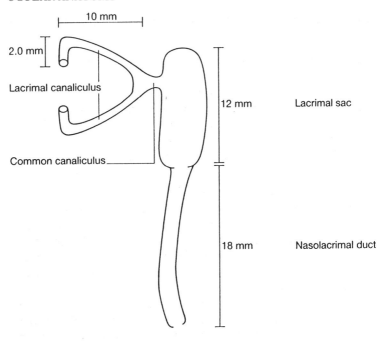

Fig 5 The lacrimal drainage system

2.5 *Lacrimal sac and nasolacrimal duct*

> a. The lacrimal sac lies in a fossa bound solely by the lacrimal bone
> b. The sac is surrounded by a fascial sheath
> c. The sac is lined by columnar cells
> d. The nasolacrimal duct is membranous
> e. The nasolacrimal duct passes downwards backwards and medially

The lacrimal sac lies in the lacrimal fossa formed by the lacrimal bone, the frontal process of maxilla, and the lacrimal fascia. The sac is covered by a fascial sheath only between the anterior and posterior lacrimal crests and is separated from the sac by a venous plexus. The lacrimal sac is lined by columnar cells and is continuous with the nasolacrimal duct. The duct is a membranous structure that passes downwards, backwards and laterally in an osseous canal to enter the inferior meatus of the nose.

2.6 Relations of the lacrimal sac and nasolacrimal duct

a. The medial palpebral ligament lies anterior to the lacrimal sac
b. The lacrimal sac lies lateral to the ethmoidal air cells
c. The angular vein lies anterior to the lacrimal sac
d. The nasolacrimal duct is formed by the maxilla and the lacrimal bone
e. The nasolacrimal duct opens into the inferior meatus

The lacrimal sac has a number of important relations, which must be considered in procedures such as dacryocystorrhinostomies. The medial palpebral ligament (lying anterior to the sac) may be divided in this procedure but care should be taken to avoid another important anterior relation—the angular vein, which lies 8 mm medial to the medial canthus. A new passageway to the nasal cavity is created by removing the thin lamina papyrecia of the ethmoidal air cells lying medial to the sac. The osseous canal for the nasolacrimal duct is formed by the maxilla, the lacrimal bone, and the inferior nasal concha; it opens into the inferior meatus of the nose.

3: The eyelids

3.1 Orbital septum and tarsal plates

a. The orbital septum is continuous with the periosteum at the orbital margins
b. The orbital septum lies anterior to the medial but posterior to the lateral palpebral ligaments
c. The upper tarsal plate measures 5 mm centrally
d. The medial palpebral ligament connects the tarsi to the anterior lacrimal crest
e. The lateral palpebral raphe connects the tarsi to the marginal tubercle

The orbital septum is continuous with the periosteum at the orbital margins and is "buttonholed" centrally to form the palpebral fissure. Above and below the palpebral fissure the septum is thickened, forming upper and lower tarsal plates. The upper tarsal plate measures 10 mm centrally and the lower tarsal plate 5 mm. Both are connected to the anterior lacrimal crest by the medial palpebral ligament and to the marginal tubercle by the lateral palpebral ligament. The lateral palpebral raphe lies anterior to the ligament and consists of interlacing fibres from the palpebral part of orbicularis oculi.

3.2 Eyelid structure

a. Meibomian glands lie within the tarsal plates
b. Meibomian glands open behind the lash follicles
c. The neurovascular plane lies between the orbicularis oculi and the tarsal plates
d. The grey line is the junction between the conjunctiva and the keratinised skin epithelium
e. The glands of Möll are modified sebaceous glands

In cross section the eyelids are seen to be made up of a number of layers (running from superficial to deep): skin, subcutaneous tissue, striated muscle fibres of the orbicularis oculi, neurovascular bundle, the orbital septum tarsal plates, and the conjunctiva. The Meibomian glands are embedded in thin tarsal plates and number approximately 35 in the upper lid and 25 in the lower lid. These glands (which produce a sebaceous secretion) open behind the lash follicles, whereas the sebaceous glands of Zeis open into each follicle. The glands of Möll are modified sweat glands. The conjunctiva becomes continuous with the keratinised skin epithelium along the posterior margins of the tarsal gland openings and not at the grey line, which lies anterior to these openings. The grey line marks the tissue plane along which a surgeon can split the eyelid into an anterior portion consisting of skin, subcutaneous tissue and muscle, and a posterior portion consisting of the tarsal plates and conjunctiva.

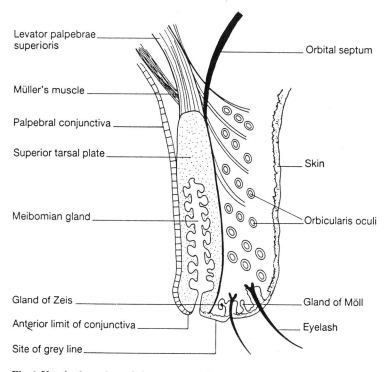

Fig 6 **Vertical section of the upper eyelid**

3.3 *Levator function*

a. The aponeurosis inserts only into the tarsal plates
b. Müller's muscle arises from the superior aspect of the levator muscle
c. The levator in an adult can raise the lid by approximately 15 mm
d. The levator palpebrae superioris is innervated by an oculomotor nerve branch passing through the superior rectus
e. Müller's muscle is innervated by sympathetic fibres from the superior cervical ganglion

11

The levator palpebrae superioris originates above the tendinous ring and passes forward above the superior rectus before fanning out into a broad aponeurosis. The bulk of the aponeurosis descends into the upper lid behind the orbital septum, which it pierces before attaching to the superior tarsal plate. Some additional fibres pass forward between the fibres of orbicularis oculi and attach to the skin to form the primary lid crease. The muscle is innervated by a branch of the oculomotor nerve, which innervates and then passes through the superior rectus en route to the levator. In the normal adult the levator is able to raise the upper lid by approximately 15 mm. The levator is assisted by Müller's muscle, which arises from the inferior aspect of the aponeurosis. This smooth muscle is inserted into the upper edge of the superior tarsal plate and is innervated by sympathetic fibres arising from the superior cervical ganglion.

3.4 Orbicularis oculi

a. Is a second branchial arch structure
b. The orbital portion is responsible for reflex blinking
c. The palpebral part extends from the medial palpebral ligament to the lateral palpebral ligament
d. The palpebral part lies in front of the orbital septum
e. The orbital part is involved in the lacrimal pump

Orbicularis oculi is a muscle of facial expression that is derived from the second branchial arch and is therefore supplied by a branch of the facial nerve. The palpebral part of the muscle that lies on either side of the palpebral fissure extends from the medial palpebral ligament to the lateral palpebral raphe. It lies in front of the orbital septum and, because of its intimate involvement with the lacrimal canaliculi, is involved in the pumping action of tears from the conjunctiva to the lacrimal sac. The palpebral portion of the muscle is also responsible for reflex blinking (as opposed to the orbital portion, which "screws" the eyelids tightly together).

3.5 Blood supply, lymphatic drainage and innervation

a. The upper eyelids are supplied by branches of the ophthalmic artery
b. Anastomoses between the internal and external carotid systems exist in the eyelids
c. Venous drainage medially is via ophthalmic and angular veins
d. Lymph from the lateral two-thirds of the upper and lower lids passes to the submandibular nodes
e. Nerves from the ophthalmic and maxillary divisions of the trigeminal innervate the lower lid

The lateral palpebral arteries (derived from the lacrimal artery) and the medial palpebral arteries (arising from the ophthalmic artery) are the main arterial supplies to the eyelids. Most of the venous drainage passes medially to the ophthalmic and angular veins, the lateral aspects draining into the superficial temporal vein. Anastomoses between the facial artery (derived from the external carotid) and the palpebral arteries (derived from the internal carotid) are present at the lateral aspect of the eyelids. Lymph from the lateral two-thirds of the upper and lower lids drains to the superficial parotid nodes; more medial lymphatic drainage is to the submandibular nodes. The lower lid receives most of its innervation from the infraorbital division of the maxillary nerve but its medial aspect is supplied by the infratrochlear nerve, a branch of the ophthalmic division of the trigeminal nerve.

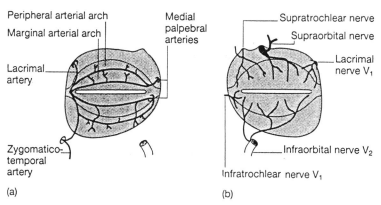

Peripheral arterial arch
Marginal arterial arch
Lacrimal artery
Zygomatico-temporal artery

Medial palpebral arteries

Supratrochlear nerve
Supraorbital nerve
Lacrimal nerve V_1
Infraorbital nerve V_2
Infratrochlear nerve V_1

(a)   (b)

Fig 7 (a) Blood supply to the eyelids. (b) Innervation of the eyelids

13

4: The conjunctiva

4.1 *Structure*

a. The palpebral conjunctiva adheres firmly to the tarsal plates
b. The fornical conjunctiva is attached to the fascial expansions of the extraocular muscle sheaths
c. The bulbar conjunctiva is closely attached to the sclera
d. The lateral fornix extends posteriorly to the equator
e. The conjunctival limbus lies 1 mm posterior to the sclerocorneal limbus

The conjunctiva may be divided in anatomical terms into palpebral and bulbar components, which are continuous at the fornices. The palpebral conjunctiva is firmly adherent to the tarsal plates. The fornical conjunctiva is attached to the fascial expansions of the extraocular muscle sheaths, allowing the conjunctiva to be drawn upwards or downwards as the recti contract. The superior fornix is situated 10 mm from the limbus and the inferior 8 mm from the limbus. The lateral fornix extends 14 mm from the limbus, passing posteriorly to the equator of the globe. The bulbar conjunctiva lies loosely over the sclera and joins with the corneal epithelium 1 mm anterior to the sclerocorneal limbus.

4.2 *Blood supply and innervation*

a. The tarsal conjunctiva is mostly supplied by the medial and lateral palpebral arteries
b. The limbal conjunctiva is supplied by branches of the anterior ciliary arteries
c. Conjunctival vessels cannot be constricted by topical adrenaline
d. Conjunctival veins may drain directly into the superior or inferior ophthalmic veins
e. The bulbar conjunctiva is innervated by the long ciliary nerves

The medial and lateral palpebral arteries divide to form marginal and peripheral arcades in both lids and are the main blood supply to the palpebral conjunctiva. The peripheral bulbar conjunctiva is supplied by branches from the peripheral arcade but the limbal conjunctiva is supplied mainly by branches from the anterior ciliary arteries. As these vessels lie superficially they will, unlike the episcleral vessels, be constricted by topical adrenaline. Conjunctival veins may drain directly into the superior or inferior ophthalmic veins; this explains their gross dilation in conditions such as cavernous sinus thrombosis. The bulbar conjunctiva is innervated by the long ciliary nerves, which are branches of the nasociliary division of the ophthalmic nerve.

4.3 *Histology*

a. The conjunctiva is a mucous membrane
b. The bulbar epithelium is stratified squamous
c. The lamina propria forms papillae at the limbus
d. Goblet cells are most common on the tarsal conjunctiva
e. Accessory lacrimal glands are found in the bulbar conjunctiva

The conjunctiva is a mucous membrane consisting of an epithelium and underlying lamina propria. The stratified squamous epithelium of the palpebral conjunctiva becomes a stratified columnar layer in the bulbar region before again becoming stratified squamous in continuation with the corneal epithelium. Another change found at the limbus is that papillae are formed by the lamina propria. The goblet cells of the conjunctiva responsible for the inner layer of the tear film are most commonly found at the inferonasal aspect of the bulbar conjunctiva, as are the accessory lacrimal glands of Krause and Wolfring.

5: The cornea

5.1 Corneal embryology

> a. Development of the cornea precedes separation of the lens cup from surface ectoderm
> b. The corneal stroma is derived from the surface ectoderm
> c. The epithelium and endothelium are derived from the surface ectoderm `
> d. The corneal diameter is determined by the optic cup diameter
> e. The fetal cornea is transparent

Corneal development begins at day 33 of gestation, after the lens cup has separated from the surface ectoderm. The corneal epithelium is derived from surface ectoderm, whereas the endothelium and fibroblasts that produce the corneal stroma are derived from neural crest cells. The final diameter of the cornea is determined by the diameter of the optic cup. The fetal cornea is very hydrated compared to the adult form and is therefore translucent rather than transparent.

5.2 Milestones in corneal development

> a. The stroma is the first layer to develop
> b. The endothelium is initially a bilayered structure
> c. Descemet's membrane is present at 3 months' gestation
> d. Corneal nerves are present at 5 months
> e. The adult form of the cornea is present at 5 months

The initial step in corneal development is the production of a bilayered epithelium and basement membrane separate from a bilayer (or occasionally a trilayer) of endothelial cells and associated basement membrane. At approximately 7 weeks' gestation a primitive stroma is formed, which is infiltrated by fibroblasts producing collagen fibrils. By the third month the stroma is a stucture of 25–30 layers, a thin Descemet's membrane is present and the endothelium is now a single layer. By 5 months the corneal nerves are present and at 7 months the cornea has reached its adult form.

5.3 Gross structure

a. The vertical diameter of the cornea is greater than its horizontal diameter
b. The anterior radius of curvature is greater than the posterior radius of curvature
c. The cornea is more curved in the vertical meridian
d. The central region of the cornea is 1 mm thick
e. The cornea's refractive index is 1.36

The cornea does not form a perfect sphere, as its average horizontal diameter (11.7 mm) is greater than its average vertical diameter (10.6 mm). The radius of curvature of the anterior surface of the cornea is approximately 7.8 mm whereas that of the posterior surface is 6.5 mm. As a rule the vertical meridian is more curved than the horizontal. The cornea measures 1.1 mm at the limbus and thins to 0.5 mm centrally. The refractive index of the cornea is 1.36 (as opposed to the aqueous humour, which has a refractive index of 1.33).

5.4 Fine structure

a. The cornea is a five-layered structure
b. The corneal epithelium is approximately 10 cells thick at the limbus
c. Bowman's layer is the basement membrane of the epithelium
d. Corneal stroma accounts for approximately 60% of total corneal thickness
e. Descemet's membrane is the basement membrane of the endothelium

The cornea is a five-layered structure consisting of an epithelium, Bowman's membrane, the stroma (or substantia propria), Descemet's membrane and an endothelium. The epithelium is a stratified structure whose superficial cells are flat and become more columnar in the deeper layers. Centrally the epithelium consists of five layers of cells, but this may increase to ten at the limbus. Bowman's layer is an acellular layer consisting of interwoven collagen fibres but it is not the basement membrane of the epithelium. Corneal stroma, made up of collagen fibres arranged in a regular lattice, account for 90% of the total corneal thickness. Descemet's membrane, which is made of collagen fibres arranged in hexagonal pattern, is the basement membrane of the endothelium.

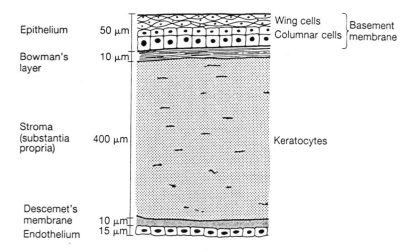

Fig 8 Fine structure of the cornea

5.5 Epithelium and endothelium

a. Both layers have microvilli
b. Basal cells of the epithelial and endothelial layers are columnar
c. Adjacent cells are linked by hemidesmosomes
d. Epithelial and endothelial cells are capable of regeneration
e. Both layers are continuous with the conjunctiva

The corneal epithelium is a multilayered structure but the endothelium is composed of a single layer of cells. The basal epithelial cells of the epithelium are columnar; the endothelial cells are cuboidal. Both surface epithelial and endothelial cells possess microvilli. Adjacent cells in both layers are linked by desmosomes; hemidesmosomes connect the cells to their respective basement membranes. Only the corneal epithelium is capable of regeneration, which occurs at the limbus with migration of epithelial cells to cover any defect. The corneal epithelium is continuous with that of the conjunctiva and the endothelium continues as a lining to the passageways of the trabecular meshwork.

5.6 Corneal innervation

a. Innervation is via the long ciliary nerves
b. The annular plexus consists of myelinated fibres
c. Fibres travel in the stroma before piercing Bowman's layer
d. Intraepithelial nerves are unmyelinated
e. The cornea is sensitive to pain, heat and cold

The cornea is predominantly innervated by the long ciliary nerves, which are branches of the ophthalmic division of the trigeminal nerve. They initially form an annular plexus of myelinated fibres at the corneal limbus with radial branches extending from this plexus in the corneal stroma to form a subepithelial plexus. Divisions from this plexus pierce Bowman's layer to form an intraepithelial plexus of unmyelinated nerves. Cold and pain are the only stimuli of the corneal epithelium.

19

5.7 *Corneal limbus*

a. The cornea becomes continuous with the sclera at the corneal limbus
b. The surgical limbus lies slightly anterior to the anatomical limbus
c. The corneal limbus lies 1 mm posterior to the conjunctival limbus
d. The endothelium forms the palisades of Vogt at the limbus
e. The groove on the inner surface of the corneal limbus contains the trabecular meshwork

The limbus or corneoscleral junction measures 1.5–2 mm in width and is the point at which the cornea becomes continuous with the sclera (this is 1 mm posterior to the conjunctival limbus). The anatomical limbus is defined by Schwalbe's line and lies slightly posterior to the surgical limbus. The outer surface is marked by a similar groove (the internal scleral sulcus) that contains the trabecular meshwork and the canal of Schlemm. The palisades of Vogt are formed by epithelial cells, which are thrown into folds by the subepithelial connective tissue at the limbus.

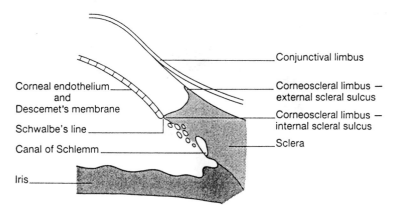

Fig 9 The corneoscleral limbus and associated structures

5.8 *Angle anatomy*

> a. Schwalbe's line marks the end of Descemet's membrane
> b. The endothelium is continuous with cells lining the trabecular meshwork
> c. Schlemm's canal lies within the internal scleral sulcus
> d. Schlemm's canal is directly connected to trabecular meshwork passages
> e. The scleral spur lies posterior to Schlemm's canal

Schwalbe's line marks the end of Descemet's membrane and the trabecular meshwork begins just posterior to this. The trabecular meshwork is attached to the scleral spur, which also contains the canal of Schlemm. The passageways of the trabecular meshwork are lined with endothelium but they are not in direct communication with the canal of Schlemm and aqueous is thought to pass between the two in giant vacuoles found in the cytoplasm of the endothelial cells.

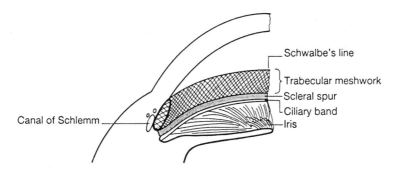

Fig 10 Gonioscopic view of a normal angle

6: The ciliary body

6.1 *Embryology*

a. The ciliary epithelium is derived from neuroectoderm
b. Epithelial differentiation occurs at 4–6 months of gestation
c. Ciliary processes are formed at 3 months
d. The primitive ciliary muscle is visible at 2 months
e. The scleral spur is fully developed at term

The ciliary body is derived from neuroectoderm and mesenchyme. The ciliary epithelium is formed from the anterior edge of the optic cup but does not differentiate like the rest of the retina. At approximately 3 months' gestation this epithelium is thrown into folds, forming the ciliary processes, and from the fourth to sixth differentiation occurs to produce tight junctions and interdigitations. The ciliary stroma is formed from mesenchyme lying between the optic cup and the cornea, with primitive muscle becoming visible at 3 months. During the fourth month a primitive scleral spur appears which is not fully formed until after the first year of life.

6.2 *Ciliary body structure*

a. The ciliary body consists of the ciliary stroma, epithelium, and muscle
b. It is continuous with the choroid posteriorly at the pars plicata
c. The ciliary body is continuous anteriorly with the peripheral iris
d. Ciliary processes arise from the pars plana
e. The lens zonule attaches to the ciliary processes

The ciliary body is a circular structure composed of the ciliary stroma, a bilayered epithelium and the ciliary muscle. It is continuous with the choroid posteriorly at the pars plana and with the peripheral iris anteriorly. The ciliary processes found at the pars plicata are regions of epithelium that have been thrown into folds and form the attachments for the zonular fibres of the lens.

6.3 Ciliary epithelium

a. The ciliary epithelium is a bilayered cuboidal epithelium
b. The inner layer is pigmented
c. The outer layer cells are rich in golgi apparatus and rough endoplasmic reticulum
d. The two cell layers lie apex to apex
e. The basement membrane of the inner layer is continuous with the basement membrane of the retinal pigment epithelium

The ciliary epithelium is a bilayered cuboidal epithelium that forms an integral part of the blood aqueous barrier. The two cell layers lie apex to apex, the inner layer being rich in golgi apparatus and rough endoplasmic reticulum while the outer layer contains numerous melanocytes. There are numerous tight junctions between the cells of the inner layer but not between cells of the two layers. The basement membrane of the inner layer is continuous with the internal limiting membrane of the retina, whereas the basement membrane of the outer layer is continuous with that of the retinal pigment epithelium.

6.4 Ciliary muscle

a. This is a striated muscle
b. Longitudinal fibres run posteriorly into the choroidal stroma
c. Oblique fibres radiate out from the scleral spur
d. The circular fibres are the most external
e. Contraction increases the refractive power of the lens

The ciliary muscle makes up the bulk of the ciliary body. It is a smooth muscle which can be divided into longitudinal, oblique and circular fibres. The longitudinal fibres run posteriorly and are attached to the choroidal stroma which therefore moves anteriorly when the eye accommodates. The oblique fibres radiating from the scleral spur increase the facilitation of aqueous outflow when they contract. The circularly arranged fibres are the most internal and their contraction slackens the tension in the zonular fibres, increasing the refractive power of the lens.

7: The iris

7.1 *Embryology*

> a. Normal development is dependent on embryonic fissure closure
> b. The tunica vasculosa lentis contributes to the iris epithelium
> c. The posterior and anterior ciliary arteries invade the stroma at 3–4 months' gestation
> d. The iris musculature is derived from mesenchyme
> e. The central pupillary membrane absorption occurs at 6 months

Normal iris development is dependent on the closure of the embryonic fissure which occurs on days 33–35; abnormal closure results in iris coloboma and/or hypoplasia. By the sixth week of development the anterior chamber boundaries have been formed by the cornea and the tunica vasculosa lentis. With the pupillary membrane the tunica vasculosa lentis will form the primitive iris stroma that is infiltrated in the third and fourth months by the long posterior and anterior ciliary arteries. During the fifth month the pupillary membrane remodels itself and at the sixth month the central portion is absorbed, forming the pupil. The sphincter and dilator muscles, and the bilayered iris epithelium, are derived from neuroectoderm.

7.2 *Muscle and epithelial development*

> a. The sphincter muscle arises from the anterior epithelial layer
> b. The dilator muscle develops before the sphincter muscle
> c. The dilator muscle develops from anterior epithelium peripheral to Von Michel's spur
> d. The dilator muscle develops from the basal processes of epithelial cells
> e. The posterior epithelium is originally pigmented

Both the iris muscle and its bilayered epithelium are derived from neuroectoderm. The sphincter and dilator muscles arise from the anterior epithelial layer. The dilator muscle develops later and is first seen as outgrowths from the basal processes of epithelial cells that lie peripheral to Von Michel's spur. The posterior epithelium does not give rise to any muscular processes and is originally unpigmented, but during the fourth month of gestation pigmentation begins at the pupil margin and spreads peripherally.

7.3 Gross structure

a. The iris consists of a posterior epithelium and an anterior stroma
b. The iris stroma is rich in melanocytes and fibroblasts
c. The collarette lies 2 mm from the pupil margin
d. The sphincter pupillae is located in the ciliary zone
e. The dilator pupillae is a radially arranged muscle

The iris is a pigmented diaphragm that consists of a posterior bilayered epithelium and an anterior stroma rich in melanocytes and fibroblasts (the colour of the iris is determined by the amount of pigment produced by the melanocytes). The collarette, which lies approximately 2 mm from the pupil margin, is the thickest region of the iris and divides it into a pupillary and ciliary zone. The sphincter pupillae is located in the pupillary zone and is a concentrically arranged muscle, whereas the dilator pupillae is arranged radially and lies in the more peripheral ciliary zone.

7.4 *Epithelium*

a. The iris epithelium is bilayered, with cells lying base to base
b. The anterior layer of iris epithelium is continuous with the outer pigmented layer of the ciliary epithelium
c. The anterior layer is rich in melanocytes
d. The positive layer is closely related to the muscular processes of the dilator muscle
e. The iris epithelium does not extend on to the anterior iris surface

The iris epithelium is a bilayered cuboidal epithelium which, like that of the ciliary body, is arranged with cells lying apex to apex. The anterior layer (which is continuous with the outer pigmented layer of the ciliary epithelium) is lacking in melanocytes, unlike the posterior layer which is heavily pigmented. The basal processes of the anterior epithelial cells give rise to the myoepithelial cells of the dilator muscle. The pigmented posterior epithelium will extend anteriorly a short distance to the ruff but any further excursion is classified as ectropion uvae.

7.5 *Blood supply of iris and ciliary body*

a. The major arterial arcade is formed solely by the long posterior ciliary arteries
b. The major arterial arcade lies in the ciliary stroma
c. The minor arcade is formed at the ruff
d. All vessels are non-fenestrated with endothelial tight junctions
e. Venous drainage is via the vortex veins

The major arterial arcade, which is formed by the long posterior ciliary arteries with communication from the anterior ciliary arteries, is the major blood supply to the iris and ciliary body. This arcade lies in the ciliary stroma and its radial branches form a further minor arcade at the collarette of the iris. Iridial vessels are non-fenestrated, with endothelial tight junctions but those vessels located in the ciliary body have numerous fenestrations and no tight junctions, the blood–aqueous barrier in this region being maintained by the tight junctions of the ciliary epithelium. The veins follow the arteries and form a minor venous circle that drains directly into the vortex veins, not into a corresponding major circle.

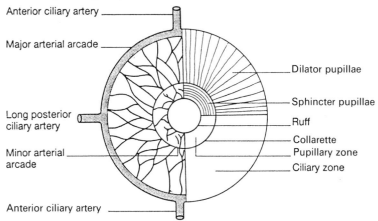

Fig 11 The iris: zones, musculature and blood supply

7.6 *Innervation of ciliary and iris muscles*

a. Parasympathetic nerves supply the ciliary muscle and sphincter pupillae

b. Parasympathetic fibres arise from the Edinger-Westphal nucleus

c. Preganglionic parasympathetic fibres travel in the short ciliary nerves

d. Long ciliary nerves carry sensory branches from the nasociliary branch of the ophthalmic division of the trigeminal nerve

e. Sympathetic fibres in the long ciliary nerves supply the dilator pupillae

Parasympathetic nerves supply the ciliary muscle and the sphincter pupillae. They arise from the Edinger-Westphal nucleus in the mid brain and travel with the oculomotor nerve to the orbit, where they synapse in the ciliary ganglion. Postganglionic fibres travel in the short ciliary nerves to supply the ciliary and sphincter muscles. The long ciliary nerves are mixed nerves containing sensory fibres from the nasociliary nerve and sympathetics from the internal carotid plexus that supply the dilator muscle.

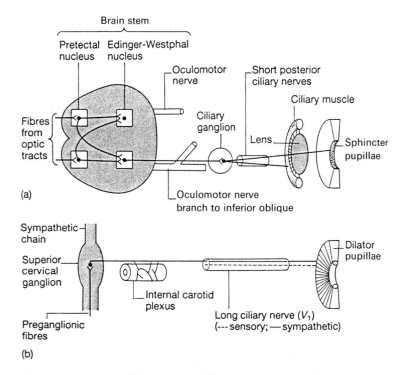

Fig 12 Innervation of the iris and ciliary muscles: (a) parasympathetic supply; (b) sympathetic supply

8: The lens

8.1 *Embryology*

a. A lens placode is formed from the surface ectoderm
b. The lens vesicle is formed at two months of gestation
c. Primary lens fibres arise from the anterior lens vesicle
d. Secondary lens fibres arise from anterior epithelial cells
e. The anteroposterior diameter of the fetal lens is initially greater than the equatorial diameter

The lens is formed from a disc shaped thickening of the surface ectoderm overlying the optic vesicle on day 27 of development. This is known as the lens placode. Substances from the optic vesicle are thought to induce placode cells to elongate so forming the lens vesicle on day 33. Cells from the posterior part of the vesicle lengthen, to form primary lens fibres that fill the vesicle lumen. The secondary lens fibres arise from the anterior epithelial cells, and migrate and taper to form the characteristic Y shaped (anterior) and inverted Y shaped (posterior) sutures. Initially the anteroposterior diameter of the fetal lens is greater than the equatorial diameter, but this situation slowly reverses.

8.2 *Gross structure*

a. The lens has a uniform capsule
b. The lens is surrounded by a cuboidal epithelium ·
c. The fetal nucleus is the innermost nucleus
d. The lens continues to grow throughout life
e. Zonular fibres run from the ciliary processes to the lens equator

The lens is a transparent biconvex structure that in the adult measures approximately 10 mm in diameter and 4 mm thick. It is surrounded by an elastic capsule, which is relatively thickened in the periequatorial regions and thinned at the anterior and posterior poles. The lenticular epithelium, which lies below the capsule, is found only on the anterior surface of the lens and is cuboidal in nature, becoming columnar as the cells approach the equator. The embryonic nucleus is the innermost nucleus of the lens and is surrounded by the fetal and adult nuclei. The epithelial cells have increased mitotic activity at the lens equator, the elongating cells becoming lens fibres and run from the posterior to the anterior lens surface. This process continues throughout life, increasing the size of the lens. Acellular fibres known as zonules connect the lens equator to the ciliary processes.

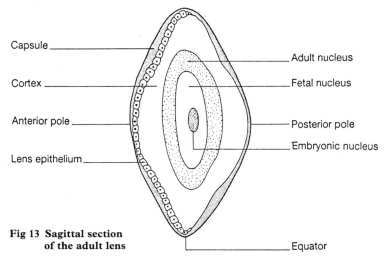

Fig 13 Sagittal section of the adult lens

8.3 *Histology*

a. Lens fibres are derived from epithelial cells
b. Mitotic activity is maximal at the anterior pole
c. The lens bow is formed by anterior migration of lens fibre nuclei
d. The anterior suture is an inverted Y shape
e. The lens cortex contains newly formed fibres

The lens fibres are formed by the mitotic activity of the epithelial cells, which is greatest at the lens equator. The maturing fibres stretch from the posterior to the anterior surface of the lens, and the migration of their nuclei anteriorly forms a characteristic lens bow. In the fetal nucleus the opposing lens fibres in the same layer produce patterns known as sutures, the anterior sutures being Y shaped and the posterior sutured an inverted Y. The lens cortex refers to the region surrounding the adult nucleus and contains the recently formed nucleated fibres.

9: The choroid and sclera

9.1 *Embryology*

a. The choroid and sclera are of mesenchymal origin
b. Choroidal development is dependent on a vascular framework
c. Choroidal melanoblasts are derived from the neural crest
d. Scleral development proceeds in a posterior to anterior direction
e. The scleral spur is fully formed at 3 months gestation

The choroid and sclera are formed by differentiation of mesenchyme surrounding the optic cup. Choroidal development is dependent on the vascular framework that develops around the long and short posterior ciliary arteries. Melanoblasts from the neural crest invade the choroidal mesenchyme during the seventh month, mature and form melanocytes. Scleral development proceeds in a posterior direction and is characterised by the laying down of collagen and elastic fibres by fibroblasts. By 3 months gestation the optic nerve is reached and by 5 months the scleral spur is fully formed.

9.2 *Choroid*

a. The choroid is part of the uveal tract
b. Choroid is firmly attached to the sclera at the optic nerve and point at which the vortex veins exit
c. Blood supply is solely from the posterior ciliary arteries
d. Choroidal capillaries are most dense at the macula
e. It is innervated by the long and short ciliary nerves

The uveal tract is a vascular pigmented layer that consists of the choroid, ciliary body and the iris. Anatomically the choroid can be divided into the vessel layer, capillary layer and Bruch's membrane. It is firmly attached to the sclera at the optic nerve and at the exit of the vortex veins. The blood vessels and the nerves supplying the choroid are found in the potential space between the choroid and the sclera (the perichoroidal space). The two posterior ciliary arteries and the short posterior ciliary artery are the main supply to the choroid but the anterior ciliary vessels also contribute. The choroidal capillaries are lined by a continuous layer of fenestrated endothelial cells and are found to be most dense at the macula (in a central retinal artery occlusion the blood flow in these vessels enables them to be seen as the characteristic foveal cherry red spot). The choroid is innervated by the long and short ciliary nerves.

9.3 *Bruch's membrane*

Bruch's membrane:
a. Measures 2–4 mm thick
b. Has the basement membrane of retinal pigment epithelial cells forming its inner layer
c. Has a bilayer of collagen
d. Lies adjacent to the vessel layer of the choroid
e. Forms part of the blood–retina barrier

Bruch's membrane is the innermost layer of the choroid and is approximately 2–4 mm in thickness. It is a five-layered structure consisting of the basement membrane of the capillary endothelium, a meshwork of elastic fibres sandwiched between a bilayer of collagen and the inner basement membrane of the retinal pigment epithelial cells. The membrane lies adjacent to the capillary layer of the choroid and does not contribute to the retinal barrier, which at this point is represented by tight junctions between the retinal pigment epithelial cells.

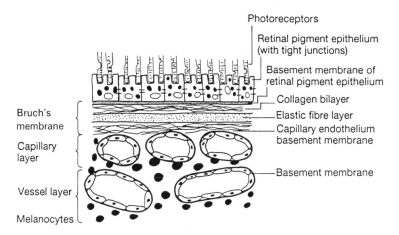

Fig 14 Schematic diagram of Bruch's membrane

9.4 *Sclera*

The sclera:
a. Is thickest posteriorly and thinnest at the equator
b. Is fused with the dural sheaths of the optic nerve
c. Forms the lamina cribrosa
d. Is pierced by the vortex veins 4 mm anterior to the equator
e. Is directly continuous with the cornea anteriorly

The sclera forms the tough relatively avascular "outer coating" of the eye, which fuses posteriorly with the dural sheaths of the optic nerve and is directly continuous with cornea anteriorly. It is thickest (1 mm) at its posterior pole, thins to 0.6 mm at the equator and is thinnest (0.3 mm) immediately posterior to the tendinous insertions of the recti. The sclera is perforated 3 mm medial and 1 mm above the posterior pole by the optic nerve: here it has a sievelike appearance and is known as the lamina cribrosa. The sclera is pierced by three other groups of structures: the anterior ciliary arteries, the long and short ciliary nerves and vessels, and the vortex veins 4 mm posterior to the equator.

9.5 *Histology*

a. The episclera is connected to Tenon's capsule
b. The episclera is relatively avascular
c. The stromal collagen is organised in a regular lattice
d. The lamina fusca contains melanocytes
e. The lamina fusca is completely separate from the choroid

The sclera consists of three layers—the episclera, the scleral stroma and the lamina fusca. The episclera consists of loose connective tissue and has a rich blood supply from the anterior ciliary arteries that lie deep to the conjunctival vessels and are not constricted by topical adrenaline. The episclera is also connected to Tenon's capsule (the fascial sheath of the eyeball). The stromal collagen is not organised in a regular lattice and is therefore not transparent. The innermost layer (the lamina fusca) contains a number of melanocytes and has some collagen connections with the overlying choroid.

10: The retina

10.1 *Formation of the optic vesicle and optic cup*

> a. The optic vesicle is an outgrowth from the mesencephalon
> b. The optic vesicle is usually formed by day 25 of gestation
> c. Involution of optic cup and stalk occurs at around 5 weeks
> d. Optic fissure closure proceeds from the cup to the forebrain
> e. The hyaloid artery is enclosed in the optic fissure during weeks 5–7

The optic vesicle is formed by a lateral out-pouching from the diencephalon and is usually fully formed by day 25. The proximal portion of the optic vesicle becomes constricted to form the optic stalk, and the dilated distal segment forms the optic cup; both become involuted during the fifth week producing a groove on their inferior aspects (known as the optic or choroidal fissure). The hyaloid artery and surrounding vascular mesenchyme are enclosed in the optic fissure. The optic cup closes in the fifth week, followed by closure of the optic stalk that proceeds from the forebrain towards the cup in week six.

10.2 *Optic vesicle*

> a. The outer layer contains pigmented pseudostratified columnar cells
> b. The inner layer has an outer nuclear and inner marginal zone
> c. Mitosis in the outer layer finishes by the fifteenth week
> d. Cell differentiation is initiated in the marginal zone
> e. The cilia of the optic vesicle disappear by week seven

The optic vesicle consists of an outer and inner layer. The outer layer is composed of pseudostratified columnar cells with pigment granules being present as early as the third week of gestation; this layer will form the retinal pigment epithelium. The inner layer (which will form the neural retina) consists of an outer nuclear and inner marginal zone. Mitosis is maximal in the outer zone of the inner layer and is completed by 15 weeks, whereas the cells of the future retinal pigment epithelium continue to divide late into fetal life. As mitosis finishes differentiation begins: this is initiated in the marginal zone. The cilia found in the outer nuclear zone of the inner layer disappear by the seventh week.

10.3 *Retinal differentiation*

a. The neural epithelium normally forms an inner and outer neuroblastic layer by week seven of gestation
b. Inner neuroblastic layers give rise to amacrine and ganglion cells
c. Lamination is complete by $2\frac{1}{2}$ months into gestation
d. The photoreceptors develop from the inner marginal zone
e. The ora serrata is fully developed at 6 months' gestational age

By the seventh week of gestation the neural epithelium has separated into inner and outer neuroblastic layers. The inner layer will produce ganglion and amacrine cells whereas the outer layer gives rise to horizontal and bipolar elements. Lamination is essentially complete by $4\frac{1}{2}$ months and the ora serrata by 6 months. Photoreceptors are thought to be derived from cilia found in the outer nuclear zone.

10.4 *Neural retina*

a. The photoreceptor nuclei are found in the outer nuclear layer
b. The outer plexiform layer contains amacrine cells and bipolar cells
c. The inner nuclear layer contains ganglion cell nuclei
d. The inner plexiform layer contains synapses between ganglion and bipolar cells
e. The nerve fibre layer consists of myelinated ganglion cells

The neural retina may be divided into nine layers based on the findings of light microscopy. The rods and cones form the outermost layer and are separated from the outer nuclear layer (in which are found the photoreceptor nuclei) by the external limiting membrane. The outer plexiform layer comprises photoreceptor and bipolar axons, and the processes of the horizontal cells. The bipolar, horizontal, and amacrine cell bodies are found in the inner nuclear layer, along with the cell bodies of the Müller cells. Processes of the bipolar, amacrine, and ganglion cells are found in the inner plexiform layer. This layer is followed by a layer of ganglion cells whose unmyelinated dendrites form the penultimate nerve fibre layer. The inner limiting membrane (made from the intraconnecting foot processes of the Müller cells) is the innermost layer.

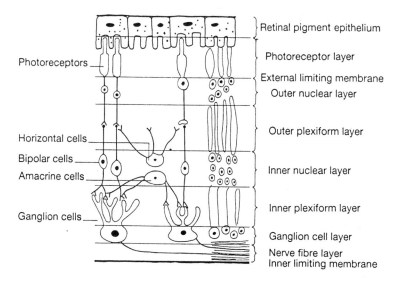

Fig 15 **The layers of the retina**

10.5 *Photoreceptors*

a. There are approximately 120 million rods in the eye
b. There are approximately 20 million cones in the eye
c. Rods are absent at the fovea
d. The ratio of photoreceptor to ganglion cells is approximately 10:1
e. Cone density decreases gradually from the fovea to the periphery

The retina contains approximately 120 million rods. They are absent from the fovea but have a maximum density of approximately 160 000/mm^2 in the perifoveal region, decreasing gradually to 30 000/mm^2 at the retinal periphery. There are approximately 6.3–6.8 million cones in the retina. They are most numerous in the rod-free fovea, and reduce to a density of 5000/mm^2 away from the fovea. Photoreceptors have a ratio with ganglion cells of 100:1.

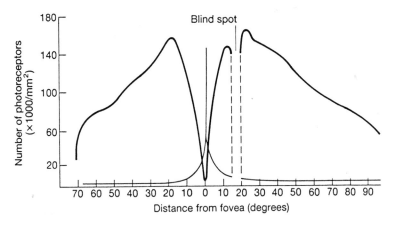

Fig 16 **Photoreceptor distribution in the retina. (—) Rods; (—) cones**

10.6 Retinal membranes and glial cells

a. Müller cells are derived from neuroectoderm
b. The inner limiting membrane is composed of Müller cell processes and their basement membranes
c. The inner limiting membrane forms part of the blood retinal barrier
d. The outer limiting membrane is formed by connections between Müller cells and retinal pigment epithelial cells
e. The outer limiting membrane forms a part of the blood retinal barrier

Müller cells are neuroglial cells and hence are derived from neuroectoderm. They are arranged radially in the retina and extend through the whole thickness of the neural retina. Their processes, in combination with their basement membranes, form the inner limiting membrane. At the outer surface of the neural retina tight junctions between photoreceptor cells and the radial processes of the Müller cells form the outer limiting membrane. Neither of these membranes contribute to the blood retinal barrier. As well as having a supportive role the Müller cells are responsible for the nutrition of retinal resources, and are responsible for the B wave of the electroretinogram.

10.7 Macular embryology

a. The macula is characterised by an increased thickness of the ganglion cell layer during the fifth month of gestation
b. Peripheral displacement of ganglion cells occurs during the seventh month
c. Cones increase in length and width during the seventh month
d. Cones are not fully developed at term
e. Ganglion cells are absent from the fovea by term

Macular development is characterised by a localised superimposition of ganglion cell nuclei at the posterior pole during the fifth month of development. By the sixth month of gestation there are eight or nine layers of nuclei but peripheral displacement of ganglion cells caused by axonal elongation commences by the seventh month. The foveal cones increase in length but decrease in width, so increasing their density, but because they are not fully developed until several months after birth the newborn infant has imperfect central fixation. At term a single layer of ganglion cells is present and an internal nuclear layer overlying the macular cones; these are displaced by the fourth month of life, leaving the central cones "uncovered".

10.8 *Macula*

a. The macula measures three disc diameters
b. The macula lies medial to the optic disc
c. The foveal floor cone concentration is approximately 100 000/mm^2
d. The foveola consists solely of photoreceptors and bipolar cells
e. The foveola is blind to the colour blue

The macula lutea is a yellowish oval area 4.5 mm (three disc diameters) long lying approximately 3 mm lateral to the optic disc. The central area of the macula is depressed and is known as the fovea centralis; it measures 1.5 mm in diameter. The cone density is maximal at this point (approximately 150 000/m^2). The floor of the fovea is known as the foveola and consists purely of photoreceptor cells, with bipolar cells being displaced peripherally. No rods are present in the foveola, rendering it blind to blue light.

10.9 *Retinal blood supply*

a. The outer two-thirds of the retina receives nutrient from the choroidal circulation
b. The central retinal artery is an end artery
c. Retinal arteries run in the nerve fibre layer
d. Retinal capillaries are absent from the fovea centralis
e. Cilioretinal arteries exist in approximately 50% of people

The outer plexiform layer is the watershed region of the retina: structures that lie peripheral to this layer (rods and cones in the outer nuclear layer) receive their nutrients by diffusion from the choroidal circulation, whereas the inner two-thirds of the retina receive nutrients directly from the central retinal artery and its tributaries. The retinal arteries run in the nerve fibre layer and are functional end arteries with four branches supplying each quadrant of the retina. The arterioles running through the different layers of the neural retina as far as the internal nuclear layer are also devoid of anastomoses and give rise to a diffuse capillary network whose walls are lined with non-fenestrated endothelial cells. These retinal capillaries are concentrated in the macula but are absent from the fovea centralis. The cilioretinal artery (arising from a posterior ciliary artery) exists in approximately 20% of people and explains why macular function may be preserved in occlusions of the central retinal artery.

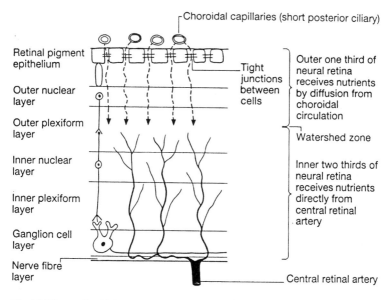

Fig 17 The retinal blood supply

11: Anterior visual pathways

11.1 Optic nerve embryology

> a. The optic stalk and cup close simultaneously
> b. All inner optic stalk cells develop vacuoles
> c. Myelination is complete by 7 weeks of gestation
> d. Meningeal sheaths are formed from neural crest mesoderm
> e. Optic nerve colobomas are usually inferotemporal

The optic nerve is formed from the primitive optic stalk. Optic stalk closure follows that of the optic cup and is dependent on breakdown of basal lamina, inversion of the outer layers of the stalk, and regeneration of the basal lamina. Cells from the inner stalk will either vacuolate to make way for ganglion cell neurones, or differentiate to form glial cells. By the seventh week of development the optic stalk is full of nerve fibres, but myelination does not commence until the seventh month. Meningeal sheaths derived from neural crest mesoderm appear in the fifth month and invest the nerve in pia, subarachnoid and dura mater. Owing to the positioning of the optic fissure, defects in its closure result in inferotemporal colobomas.

11.2 Optic nerve

> a. The optic disc measures approximately 2 mm in diameter
> b. The intraorbital portion of the optic nerve is approximately 25 mm long
> c. A sheath of dura, arachnoid and pia mater surrounds the optic nerve
> d. Ganglion cells become myelinated only posterior to the chiasma
> e. The optic canal lies wholly within the sphenoid bone

The optic nerve is part of the central nervous system and as such has a meningeal sheath of dura, arachnoid and pia mater. For descriptive purposes it may be divided into four parts: the intraocular, intraorbital, intracanalicular and intracranial portions. The intraocular portion is represented by the optic disc, which measures 1.5 mm in diameter and is the point at which the optic nerve pierces the sclera. The intraorbital portion is approximately 25 mm long—here the central retinal artery enters and the central retinal vein exits the dural sheath. The nerve chiefly comprises ganglion cell neurones, which become myelinated only posterior to the lamina cribrosa. However, it also contains a number of neuroglial cells such as astrocytes. The optic canal (which lies wholly within the lesser wing of the sphenoid bone) measures approximately 5 mm long and transmits the optic nerve and ophthalmic artery. The intracranial portion of the optic nerve travels upwards, backwards and medially to reach the optic chiasma.

11.3 *Relations of the optic nerve*

a. The ciliary ganglion lies medial to the optic nerve
b. The nasociliary nerve and ophthalmic artery cross the optic nerve superiorly
c. The central retinal artery pierces the inferomedial aspect 12 mm behind the globe
d. The optic nerve lies within the muscular cone at the orbital apex
e. It lies with the ophthalmic artery and vein in the optic canal

The optic nerve has a number of important relations in the orbit. It runs superomedial to the ophthalmic artery in the optic canal and enters the orbital apex within the muscular cone. The ophthalmic artery and nasociliary nerve pass above it from lateral to medial, the ophthalmic artery having already given off the central retinal artery. The central retinal artery passes inferior to the optic nerve and pierces the inferomedial aspect of the dural sheath 12 mm behind the globe. The ciliary ganglion lies lateral to the nerve, between it and the lateral rectus muscle.

11.4 *Optic chiasma*

The optic chiasma lies:
a. Inferior to the lamina terminalis
b. Superior to the infundibulum
c. Lateral to the internal carotid
d. Superior to the diaphragma sellae
e. Inferior to the cavernous sinus

The optic chiasma is the point at which fibres from the respective nasal retinas decussate. It lies inferior to the floor of the third ventricle, just below the lamina terminalis, and has a number of important anatomical relations. The chiasma lies superior to the diaphragma sellae (which transmits the pituitary stalk or infundibulum). Anteriorly it is related to the anterior cerebral arteries, superiorly to the anterior communicating artery, and laterally to the internal carotid artery and the cavernous sinus.

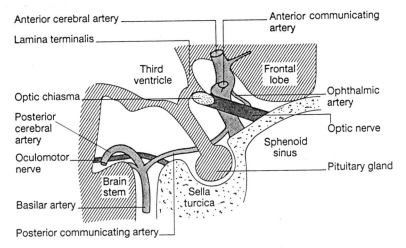

Fig 18 Relations of the optic chiasma (sagittal section)

11.5 Blood supply to the anterior visual pathway

a. The central retinal artery supplies the intraocular optic nerve
b. Short posterior ciliary arteries anastomose with the central retinal artery at the optic nerve head
c. The orbital optic nerve is primarily supplied by pial plexus vessels
d. The intracranial optic nerve is supplied by the superior hypophyseal and ophthalmic arteries
e. The optic nerve blood supply is compromised by raised intracranial pressure

The intracranial optic nerve is supplied by the superior hypophyseal and ophthalmic arteries. Despite the fact that the central retinal artery pierces the dural sheaths of the orbital optic nerve, its primary blood supply is from a pial plexus of vessels and not from the central retinal artery. The intraocular portion of the optic nerve is supplied by the short posterior ciliary arteries that form the Circle of Zinn; this forms no significant anastomoses with branches of the central retinal artery. The central retinal artery and vein run within the optic nerve's dural sheath, and a rise in intracranial pressure may compromise blood flow in these vessels (for example, the venous engorgement seen in papilloedema).

11.6 Lesions in the afferent visual pathway

a. Inferior and anterior chiasmal lesions produce superotemporal defects
b. Distal optic nerve lesions may produce bilateral field loss
c. All post chiasmal lesions produce a bilateral field defect
d. Lesion of the lateral geniculate nucleus are associated with profound ipsilateral sensory loss
e. Temporal lobe lesions tend to cause superior quadrantic field defects

A knowledge of the anatomy of the afferent visual pathway is essential when interpreting field loss secondary to lesions in the afferent visual system. The optic chiasma is the site at which fibres from the nasal retinas decussate. Fibres from the inferonasal quadrants decussate in the inferior and anterior region of the chiasma, and so lesions here will produce superotemporal field defects. These decussating fibres may pass anteriorly into the contralateral optic nerve before passing to the optic tracts and so lesions in the distal optic nerve may produce bilateral field loss. In general, post chiasma lesions will produce a homonymous hemianopia (which need not be symmetrical because chiasmal decussation is often slightly asymmetrical). An exception to this rule is a lesion found at the anterior aspect of the calcarine sulcus, which receives fibres only from the contralateral nasal retina: lesions here will produce a contralateral temporal crescentic defect. Lesions of the lateral geniculate nucleus characteristically produce contralateral hemianopias that are associated with profound contralateral sensory loss. Optic tract fibres found in the temporal lobe tend to arise from the inferior nasal and temporal quadrants, producing superior quadrantic field defects.

11.7 *Primary visual cortex*

a. The primary visual cortex is Brodmann's area 18
b. Lesions above the calcarine sulcus produce contralateral and inferior field defects
c. Macular fibres are found posteriorly
d. Superotemporal retinal fibres connect with ipsilateral cells lying above the sulcus
e. Cortical blindness is characterised by absent pupillary reflexes

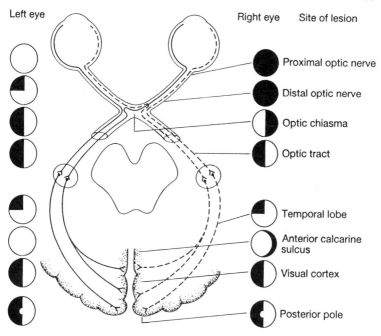

Fig 19 Visual field deficits

The primary visual cortex is situated in the walls of the calcarine sulcus found in the medial aspect of the cerebral hemisphere. It extends from the junction of the calcarine and parieto-occipital sulci to the occipital pole posteriorly and is Brodmann's area 17. The area above the calcarine sulcus receives information from the contralateral and inferior visual field via ipsilateral supero-temporal fibres and contralateral superonasal fibres. The macula, which has a relatively large representation in the visual cortex, is located at the posterior aspect of the calcarine sulcus and extends to the posterior lateral aspect of the occipital lobe. Cortical blindness, which results from infarction of the primary visual cortex, is often denied by the patient and is characterised by normal pupillary reflexes.

11.8 *Blood supply to the optic tracts and cortex*

a. The anterior choroidal and posterior communicating arteries supply the optic tracts
b. The lateral geniculate nucleus is supplied by the anterior communicating artery
c. The posterior optic radiations are supplied solely by the posterior cerebral artery
d. The visual cortex is supplied primarily by the posterior cerebral artery
e. Middle and posterior cerebral anastomoses exist near the posterior pole

The optic tracts are supplied by pial arteries derived from the anterior choroidal and posterior communicating arteries, with the occasional branch from the middle cerebral artery. The lateral geniculate nucleus is supplied by the middle cerebral artery which, along with the posterior cerebral artery, supplies the posterior aspects of the optic radiations. The visual cortex derives most of its blood supply from the posterior cerebral artery but some communication with the middle cerebral artery may exist over the occipital pole and indeed may explain the phenomena of "macular sparing" seen in some occipital lobe strokes.

12: The extraocular muscles

12.1 *The rectus muscles*

a. All rectus muscles arise from the annulus of Zinn
b. Vertical recti run at approximately 25° to the optical axis
c. The lateral rectus inserts on average 7.7 mm from the limbus
d. The medial rectus inserts on average 5.5 mm from the limbus
e. The lateral rectus has the longest tendon

All rectus muscles arise from a common tendinous origin, the annulus of Zinn, which is situated at the orbital apex. All four muscles run anteriorly, the superior and inferior recti passing forwards at approximately 25° to the optical axis of the globe. The recti insert at varying distances from the corneal limbus: the medial rectus inserts 5.5 mm from the limbus; the inferior 6.5 mm; the lateral 6.9 mm; and the superior 7.7 mm (these are average, not absolute measurements). These insertions form a spiral—the Spiral of Tilau. The medial rectus has the shortest tendon (3.7 mm); that of the lateral rectus is the longest at 8.8 mm. The above measurements are of primary importance if recessions and resections of these muscles are to be considered in surgery for strabismus.

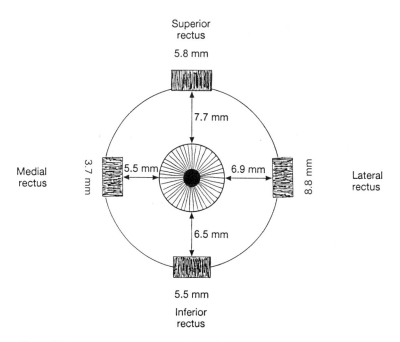

Fig 20 The rectus muscle insertions and tendon lengths of the left eye

12.2 *The oblique muscles*

> a. The superior oblique arises from the annulus of Zinn
> b. The inferior oblique arises from within the orbital rim
> c. The superior and inferior oblique muscles insert behind the equator of the globe
> d. The obliques pull at equal angles to the optical axis of the globe
> e. Both the oblique muscles pass below their corresponding rectus muscle

The superior oblique muscle arises from the body of the sphenoid bone outside the tendinous ring and gives rise to a rounded tendon that passes through the trochlea at the superonasal aspect of the orbit. The inferior oblique arises from within the floor of the orbital rim. The superior oblique pulls forward at an angle of approximately 55° to the nasal side of the globe's visual axis with the eye in the primary position; the inferior oblique pulls at an angle of approximately 50°. Both oblique muscles pass inferiorly to their corresponding rectus muscle before inserting posterior to the equator of the globe.

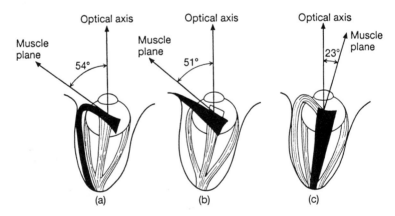

**Fig 21 Orientation of oblique and vertical recti in the primary position.
(a) Superior oblique (right, from above); (b) inferior oblique (left, from below); (c) superior rectus (right, from above)**

12.3 *Innervation*

a. The medial rectus is supplied by the inferior division of the oculomotor nerve
b. The superior rectus is the only muscle supplied by the superior division of the oculomotor nerve
c. The superior oblique is supplied by the trochlear nerve
d. The nerve to the lateral rectus enters the orbit outside the tendinous ring
e. The inferior oblique is supplied by the inferior division of the oculomotor nerve

The third cranial (or oculomotor) nerve supplies the majority of the extraocular muscles. It divides into superior and inferior divisions just before entering the orbit via the superior orbital fissure. The inferior division supplies the medial rectus, inferior rectus, and inferior oblique; the superior division supplies the superior rectus, and the levator palpebrae superioris. The superior oblique muscle is supplied by the fourth cranial nerve, the trochlear nerve. The sixth cranial (abducent) nerve, which enters the orbit through the inferior aspect of the superior orbital fissure (but within the tendinous ring), supplies the lateral rectus.

12.4 *Relations of the extraocular muscles*

a. The frontal nerve lies between the levator and superior rectus
b. The lacrimal artery and nerve lie medial to the lateral rectus
c. The abducent nerve lies lateral to the lateral rectus
d. The nasociliary nerve lies superior to the medial rectus
e. The oculomotor nerve lies superior to the inferior rectus

51

The only three nerves to enter the orbit outside the common tendinous ring are the lacrimal nerve, the frontal component of the ophthalmic nerve, and the trochlear nerve. The frontal nerve is found above the levator muscle and the lacrimal nerve (plus accompanying artery) is found superior to the lateral rectus. The nasociliary nerve, a direct continuation of the ophthalmic division of the trigeminal, passes along the superior border of the medial rectus before dividing into the anterior ethmoidal and infratrochlear nerves. The inferior division of the oculomotor nerve runs superior to the inferior rectus and medial to the abducent nerve, which lies on the medial aspect of the lateral rectus.

13: The cranial nerves

13.1 Oculomotor nerve

a. The nucleus of the oculomotor nerve lies adjacent to the inferior colliculus
b. The oculomotor nerve lies between the posterior cerebral and superior cerebellar arteries
c. It lies in the medial wall of the cavernous sinus
d. The branch to the inferior oblique carries parasympathetic fibres to the ciliary ganglion
e. The superior rectus is supplied by the contralateral oculomotor nucleus

The oculomotor nerve is the third cranial nerve and its group of nuclei are found adjacent to the superior colliculus in the mid brain. It runs anteriorly, passing the red nucleus, and emerges on the ventral surface of the mid brain to lie between the posterior cerebral and superior cerebellar arteries. Aneurysms of the posterior communicating artery, which lies parallel to the nerve, may compress it, resulting in paresis. It runs anteriorly in the lateral wall of the cavernous sinus and enters the orbit (after dividing into superior and inferior branches) via the superior orbital fissure. The oculomotor nerve supplies all the extra-ocular muscles except the lateral rectus and superior oblique; its inferior branch carries parasympathetic fibres to the ciliary ganglion. The superior rectus is the only muscle supplied by the contralateral oculomotor nucleus.

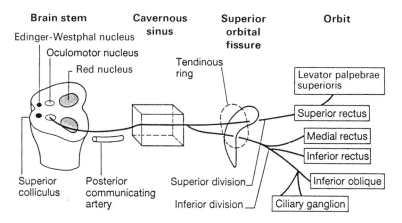

Fig 22 The oculomotor nerve

13.2 *Trochlear nerve*

a. The trochlear nerve is the only cranial nerve to exit the brain stem on its dorsal aspect
b. On leaving the cavernous sinus the trochlear nerve lies above and lateral to the oculomotor nerve
c. The trochlear nerve enters the orbit through the tendinous ring
d. The trochlear nucleus supplies the ipsilateral superior oblique
e. Damage to the trochlear nerve may result in a contralateral head tilt

The trochlear nerve is the fourth cranial nerve. Its nucleus is situated by the inferior colliculus and its fibres decussate before emerging from the dorsal aspect of the brain stem. The nerve then runs forward, travelling in the subarachnoid space around the cerebral peduncle, to enter the lateral wall of the cavernous sinus. It initially lies inferior to the oculomotor nerve but moves to lie superior and lateral to the oculomotor nerve on leaving the sinus. It enters the orbit through the superior orbital fissure outside the tendinous ring, and as the fibres decussate before leaving the brain stem it innervates the contralateral superior oblique. Damage to the trochlear nerve results in superior oblique paralysis and a contralateral head tilt.

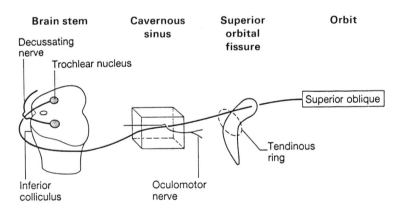

Fig 23 The trochlear nerve

13.3 *Abducent nerve*

a. The nucleus of this nerve underlies the facial colliculus
b. The abducent nerve emerges from the brain stem in the cerebellopontine angle
c. Infection of the temporal bone may damage the abducent nerve
d. This is usually the first nerve to be damaged in cavernous sinus thrombosis
e. The abducent nerve enters the orbit by passing outside the tendinous ring

The abducent nerve is the sixth cranial nerve. Its nucleus lies in the floor of the fourth ventricle, where the seventh cranial nerve passes over it (so forming the facial colliculus). It emerges from the brain stem in the cerebellopontine angle, where it may be damaged by tumours such as acoustic neuromas. It passes up the clivus in the subarachnoid space and passes over the apex of the petrous temporal bone (middle ear infection may cause abducent nerve paresis—such as Gradenigo's syndrome). The abducent nerve is the only nerve to lie in the dural walls of the cavernous sinus and therefore is often the first to be damaged by thrombosis of the sinus. It enters the orbit through the superior orbital fissure inside the common tendinous ring and pierces the lateral rectus muscle (which it supplies).

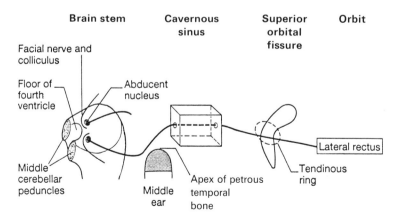

Fig 24 The abducent nerve

13.4 *Ophthalmic division of the trigeminal nerve*

a. The ophthalmic division of the trigeminal divides in the orbit to form the lacrimal, frontal and nasociliary nerves
b. The lacrimal nerve carries parasympathetic fibres from the oculomotor nerve
c. Branches supply the frontal sinus
d. The nasociliary nerve receives sensory fibres from the ciliary ganglion
e. The skin at the tip of the nose is supplied by the nasociliary nerve

The ophthalmic division of the trigeminal nerve is a purely sensory nerve that lies in the lateral wall of the cavernous sinus and divides into lacrimal, frontal, and nasociliary branches before entering the orbit. The lacrimal and frontal nerves enter the orbit outside the tendinous ring before receiving parasympathetic fibres (bound for the lacrimal gland) from the zygomaticotemporal branch of the maxillary nerve. The frontal nerve supplies the frontal sinuses via its supraorbital and supratrochlear divisions. The nasociliary nerve is the largest branch and enters the orbit through the tendinous ring. It is also the major sensory nerve to the globe, because it receives fibres from the long ciliary nerves, and from the short ciliary nerves that travel via the ciliary ganglion. The anterior ethmoidal nerve is a terminal branch of the nasociliary nerve; it supplies the lateral wall of the nose and parts of the nasal septum, and terminates on the tip of the nose as the external nasal nerve. Herpes zoster lesions affecting the tip of the nose may signal ocular involvement via the nasociliary nerves (Hutchinson's sign).

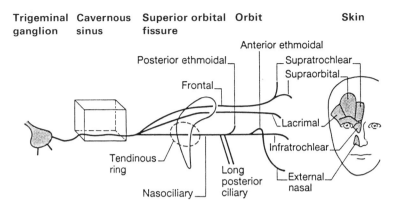

Fig 25 **The ophthalmic division of the trigeminal nerve (V1)**

13.5 *Maxillary division of the trigeminal nerve*

a. This is a purely sensory nerve
b. It lies in the lateral wall of the cavernous sinus
c. This division of the trigeminal nerve enters the infra-temporal fossa via the foramen rotundum
d. It supplies sensation to the maxillary sinus
e. Blowout fractures often cause cheek paraesthesia

The maxillary division of the trigeminal nerve is a purely sensory nerve, which, after leaving the trigeminal ganglion, lies in the lateral wall of the cavernous sinus. It then passes through the foramen rotundum and hence into the pterygopalatine fossa. It is the sensory supply to the pterygopalatine ganglion (which is suspended from the nerve) and exits the fossa as the infraorbital nerve. The infraorbital nerve, which lies in the infraorbital canal in the floor of the orbit, is responsible for the innervation of the maxillary sinuses, the upper incisor, canine, and premolar teeth, and the skin of the cheek, lower eyelid and the upper lip. "Blowout" fractures of the orbital floor often damage the nerve, causing paraesthesia in these areas.

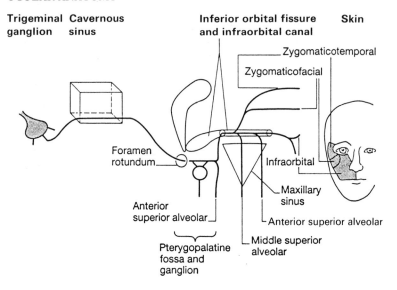

Fig 26 The maxillary division of the trigeminal nerve (V2)

14: Autonomic nervous system of the head and neck

14.1 *Sympathetic supply to the head and neck*

a. Most of the preganglionic fibres to the head and neck exit the spinal cord at T1
b. The sympathetic chain lies by the neck of the first rib
c. The sympathetic chain lies lateral to the carotid sheath
d. Head and neck fibres synapse in the superior cervical ganglion
e. Postganglionic fibres "hitchhike" on the internal carotid

Most of the preganglionic sympathetic fibres bound for the head and neck exit the spinal cord in the T1 nerve root before forming white rami communicantes to the sympathetic chain. The sympathetic chain lies by the neck of the first rib (in close proximity to the apex of the lung) and passes superiorly, lying just posteromedial to the carotid sheath. All fibres bound for the head and neck will synapse in the superior cervical ganglion, with most postganglionic fibres "hitchhiking" along the internal carotid to their destinations. Postganglionic fibres also travel on the external carotid arteries and on the third to sixth, ninth, tenth, and twelfth cranial nerves.

14.2 *Parasympathetic nuclei*

a. The Edinger-Westphal nucleus supplies fibres to the sphincter pupillae
b. The superior salivatory nucleus supplies fibres to the lacrimal gland
c. The inferior salivatory nucleus supplies fibres to the submandibular and sublingual glands
d. The superior salivatory nucleus supplies fibres to the parotid gland
e. The dorsal motor nucleus supplies fibres to the gastrointestinal tract

The parasympathetic nuclei are mid line nuclei that give rise to preganglionic myelinated fibres emerging from the brain stem with cranial nerves. The Edinger-Westphal nucleus supplies fibres that "hitchhike" with the oculomotor nerve to the ciliary ganglion and hence to the sphincter pupillae and ciliary muscles. The superior salivatory nucleus produces fibres that travel in the nervus intermedius of the seventh cranial nerve and will eventually reach the lacrimal, submandibular, sublingual, nasal, and palatal glands. The inferior salivatory nucleus is associated with the glossopharyngeal nerve and supplies fibres to the parotid gland via the otic ganglion. The dorsal motor nucleus is the secretomotor nucleus of the vagus nerve and supplies fibres to the gastrointestinal tract.

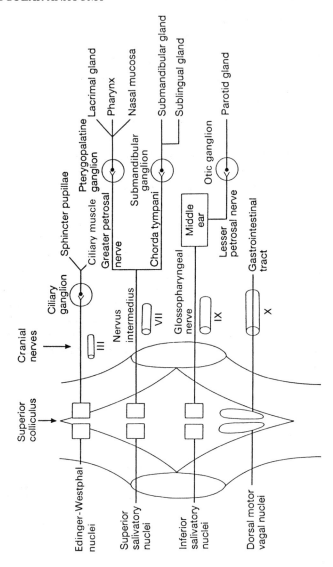

Fig 27 Parasympathetic nuclei and their connections

14.3 *Ciliary ganglion*

a. The ciliary ganglion lies lateral to the optic nerve
b. It contains parasympathetic fibres from the superior division of the oculomotor nerve, which synapse in the ganglion
c. Sympathetic fibres from the internal carotid synapse in the ganglion
d. Short ciliary nerves contain parasympathetic, sympathetic, and sensory fibres
e. Ganglion lesions may cause a tonic pupil

The ciliary ganglion is the primary autonomic ganglion of the orbit. It lies near the apex of the orbit and lateral to the optic nerve. It receives parasympathetic fibres from the inferior division of the oculomotor nerve; these are the only fibres to synapse in the ganglion. The sympathetic input is from post-ganglionic fibres travelling on the internal carotid artery. Short ciliary nerves contain parasympathetic, sympathetic, and sensory fibres. An Adie's pupil is characterised by a tonic near response and is thought to be caused by a ciliary ganglion lesion of unknown aetiology.

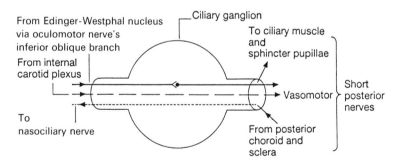

Fig 28 The ciliary ganglion. (—) Parasympathetic fibres; (- -) sympathetic fibres; (- - - -) sensory fibres

14.4 *Pterygopalatine ganglion*

a. Parasympathetic fibres travel in the greater petrosal nerve to the pterygoid canal
b. The vidian nerve is a purely parasympathetic nerve
c. The ganglion receives sensory fibres from the maxillary nerve
d. Its branches innervate the pharynx, palate, lateral nasal walls and nasal septum
e. Postganglionic fibres "hitchhike" on the zygomaticotemporal nerve, which leads them into the lacrimal gland

The pterygopalatine ganglion, like all head and neck parasympathetic ganglia, receives parasympathetic, sympathetic, and sensory fibres. The parasympathetic fibres originate from the nervus intermedius and travel in the greater petrosal nerve to the pterygoid canal where they join sympathetic fibres from the deep petrosal nerve to form the vidian nerve. Sensory fibres from the maxillary division of the trigeminal nerve pass through the ganglion and innervate the palate, nasopharynx, the lateral aspect of the nose, and parts of the nasal septum. Postganglionic parasympathetic fibres will "hitchhike" on the zygomaticotemporal branch of the maxillary nerve and then on the lacrimal nerve, before entering the lacrimal gland.

14.5 *Pupillary pathways*

a. Postgeniculate fibres synapse in the pretectal nuclei
b. The pretectal nucleus receives fibres only from the ipsilateral eye
c. Decussating fibres from pretectal nuclei pass ventral to the aqueduct
d. The Edinger-Westphal nucleus receives inputs from both eyes
e. Parasympathetic fibres "hitchhike" on the oculomotor nerve to the ciliary ganglion

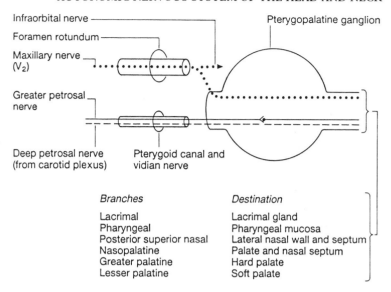

Branches	Destination
Lacrimal	Lacrimal gland
Pharyngeal	Pharyngeal mucosa
Posterior superior nasal	Lateral nasal wall and septum
Nasopalatine	Palate and nasal septum
Greater palatine	Hard palate
Lesser palatine	Soft palate

Fig 29 The pterygopalatine ganglion. (—) Parasympathetic fibres; (– –) sympathetic fibres; (· · · ·) sensory fibres

The pupillary pathway may be divided into the afferent and efferent limbs. Fibres from the optic tracts (pregeniculate fibres) synapse in the pretectal nuclei. Each pretectal nucleus will receive only an ipsilateral input, but fibres from each nucleus will connect with both the ipsilateral and contralateral Edinger-Westphal nuclei. Decussating fibres from the pretectal nuclei pass dorsal to the aqueduct. The efferent limb of the pupillary reflex consists of the preganglionic parasympathetic fibres (arising from the Edinger-Westphal nucleus) that "hitch-hike" along the oculomotor nerve to the ciliary ganglion, where they synapse and continue in the short ciliary nerves to the constrictor pupillae.

15: Orbital blood vessels and cavernous sinus

15.1 *Ophthalmic artery*

a. This is the first branch of the internal carotid after it exits the cavernous sinus
b. The ophthalmic artery lies within the dural sheath of the optic nerve in the optic canal
c. In the orbit the ophthalmic artery passes inferior to the optic nerve in 85% of people
d. It gives rise to the nasociliary artery
e. The ethmoidal and frontal sinuses are supplied by the ophthalmic artery

The ophthalmic artery is the first branch of the internal carotid as it emerges from the cavernous sinus. It lies inferolateral to the optic nerve in the optic canal and is enclosed in its dural sheath. On entering the orbit the ophthalmic artery passes above the optic nerve in 85% of cases but before doing this it gives off the central retinal artery, which passes below the nerve. Other important branches of the ophthalmic artery include the long and short posterior ciliary arteries, anterior and posterior ethmoidal arteries (which supply the ethmoidal sinuses), and the supraorbital artery (which normally supplies the frontal sinus). Its terminal branches are the supratrochlear and the dorsal nasal arteries.

15.2 *Central retinal artery*

The central retinal artery:
a. Arises from the ophthalmic artery
b. Passes superior to the optic nerve
c. Pierces the dural sheath 12 mm behind the globe
d. Supplies the pial sheath of the optic nerve
e. Is functionally an end artery

The central retinal artery arises from the ophthalmic artery where it lies inferolateral to the optic nerve. It then passes inferior to the optic nerve and pierces the dural sheath approximately 12 mm behind the globe. It travels obliquely through the subarachnoid space (accompanied by the central retinal vein) and gives off a number of small meningeal branches that supply the pial sheath of the optic nerve. Although some minute anastomoses exist between these pial branches and the short posterior ciliary arteries, the central retinal artery should be considered as an end artery.

15.3 *Ciliary arteries*

a. The long posterior ciliary arteries supply the choroid posterior to the equator
b. The long posterior ciliary arteries contribute to the major arterial circle
c. Two anterior ciliary arteries accompany each rectus muscle
d. Short posterior ciliaries supply the optic nerve head
e. Anastomoses exist between the short and the long posterior ciliary arteries

The long posterior, short posterior, and anterior ciliary arteries constitute the major blood supply to the globe. The paired long posterior ciliary arteries pierce the sclera outside the circle of Zinn and travel forward in the suprachoroidal space to the ciliary body, where they contribute to the major arterial arcade. Recurrent branches supplying the choroid anterior to the equator anastomose with the short posterior ciliaries. The short posterior ciliaries (which divide into 10–20 branches) pierce the sclera around the optic nerve; this anastomotic circle of Zinn supplies the optic nerve head, with the more anterior branches supplying the choroid as far as the equator. The anterior ciliary arteries arise from the muscular branches of the ophthalmic artery; two arteries accompany each rectus muscle (except the lateral rectus, which has only one associated artery). They supply the sclera and conjunctiva as well as contributing to the major arterial circle of the iris.

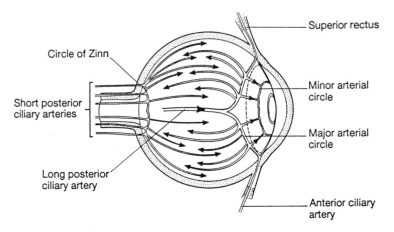

Fig 30 The ciliary arteries

15.4 *Venous drainage of the globe*

a. The superior ophthalmic vein is formed by branches of the supraorbital and facial veins
b. The vortex veins enter the superior ophthalmic vein only
c. The central retinal vein joins the superior ophthalmic vein
d. The inferior ophthalmic vein communicates with the pterygoid venous plexus
e. The inferior and superior ophthalmic veins may enter the cavernous sinus separately

The superior ophthalmic vein (usually the larger of the two ophthalmic veins) is formed by the supraorbital and facial veins. It travels posteriorly in the orbit and receives contributions from the superior vortex veins, and the central retinal vein. The inferior ophthalmic vein receives the inferior vortex veins and usually drains into the superior ophthalmic vein; it may, however, enter the cavernous sinus separately. The inferior ophthalmic vein also communicates with the pterygoid venous plexus and (as the orbital veins have no valves) spread of infection from this plexus may eventually reach the cavernous sinus, causing a cavernous sinus thrombosis.

15.5 *Connections of the cavernous sinus*

The cavernous sinus:
a. Receives blood from the sphenoparietal sinus
b. Receives the superior ophthalmic vein via the superior orbital fissure
c. Communicates with the contralateral cavernous sinus
d. Receives blood from the superior and inferior petrosal sinuses
e. Communicates with the pterygoid venous plexus via the foramen spinosum

The cavernous sinuses (which lie between the inner meningeal and outer endosteal layers of dura mater) are situated on either side of the body of the sphenoid bone. Tributaries that contribute to the cavernous sinus include the superior ophthalmic vein, part or all of the inferior ophthalmic vein, the sphenoparietal sinus (that accompanies the middle meningeal artery), and the inferior and superficial middle cerebral vein (not shown in Fig 31). Numerous interconnections exist between adjacent sinuses and drainage is predominantly via the superior and inferior petrosal sinuses and hence into the sigmoid sinus and internal jugular vein respectively. Communications also exist via emissary veins that pass through the foramen ovale or foramen of Vesalius to the pterygoid venous plexus.

15.6 *Contents and relations of the cavernous sinus*

a. The pituitary fossa lies medially
b. The greater wing of the sphenoid lies inferiorly
c. The internal carotid artery lies superiorly
d. The internal carotid artery alone lies within the cavernous sinus
e. The oculomotor, trochlear and ophthalmic division of the trigeminal are the only nerves found in its lateral wall

OCULAR ANATOMY

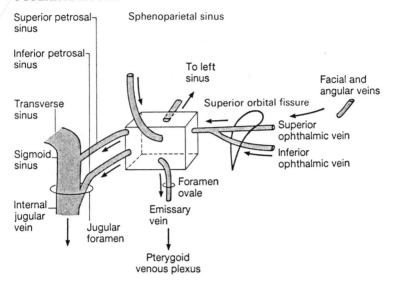

Fig 31 The major connections of the right cavernous sinus

The cavernous sinuses have a number of important contents and relations. The cavernous sinus extends from the superior orbital fissure anteriorly to the apex of the petrous part of the temporal bone posteriorly, with its floor formed by the dural coverings of the greater wing of the sphenoid bone. Lying lateral to the body of the sphenoid bone, the pituitary fossa is an important medial relation. The internal carotid artery leaves the foramen lacerum and enters the posterior part of the sinus before arching upwards and forwards, grooving the medial wall of the sinus; it eventually pierces the roof of the sinus before passing backwards towards the anterior perforate substance of the brain. The abducent nerve also travels within the cavernous sinus and is often the first structure damaged in cavernous sinus thrombosis. It should, however, be noted that both the internal carotid artery and the abducent nerve lie outside the endothelial lining of the sinus. The lateral wall of the cavernous sinus encloses the oculomotor nerve, trochlear nerve, and the first two divisions of the trigeminal nerve.

68

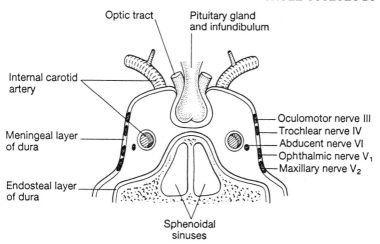

Fig 32 Contents and relations of the cavernous sinus

16: Skull osteology

16.1 *Sutures*

a. The coronal suture separates the frontal and parietal bones
b. The sagittal suture separates the parietal bones
c. Parietal and occipital bones meet at the bregma
d. The lambda is the remains of the anterior fontanelle
e. The pterion comprises the frontal, parietal, sphenoid, and temporal bones

The coronal suture extends from pterion to pterion between the frontal and the two parietal bones. The sagittal suture, which separates the parietal bones, runs from the bregma (the remains of the anterior fontanelle) anteriorly to the lambda posteriorly (the junction of the parietal bones and occipital bone). The pterion (situated approximately 3 cm above the zygomatic arch) is the meeting place of the frontal, parietal, sphenoid, and temporal bones, which usually form an H-shaped junction. This site is of topographical importance in that fractures here may rupture the middle meningeal artery (which passes through a bony canal at this point), producing an extradural haematoma.

16.2 *Sphenoid bone*

> a. This bone consists solely of greater and lesser wings plus a body
> b. The sphenoid bone articulates with the basiocciput
> c. The superior orbital fissure lies between the greater and lesser wings
> d. The foramen rotundum lies within the lesser wing of the sphenoid
> e. The pterygoid canal lies medial to the foramen rotundum

The sphenoid bone is one of the most complicated skull bones and is divided into greater and lesser wings, a body, and two pterygoid processes. The body of the sphenoid articulates with the basiocciput at a synchondrosis that fuses at the age of about 25, and is an important constituent of the skull base. The lesser wing of the sphenoid contains the optic canal and forms the boundary of the superior orbital fissure with the greater wing. The base of the pterygoid process is perforated by the foramen rotundum, which lies lateral to the smaller pterygoid canal.

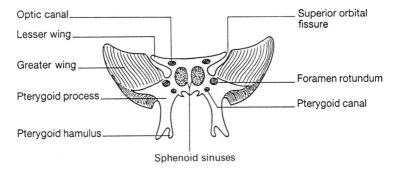

Fig 33 Frontal view of the sphenoid bone

16.3 Temporal bone

a. The temporal bone forms part of the zygomatic arch
b. The petrous part of the temporal bone houses the middle ear
c. It transmits the stylomastoid foramen
d. It transmits the jugular canal
e. Mastoid air cells are present at birth

The temporal bone may, like the sphenoid bone, be divided into a number of parts for descriptive purposes. The squamous part articulates with the greater wing of the sphenoid and the parietal bone; its zygomatic process forms part of the zygomatic arch. The petrous part houses the middle ear and labyrinth, and is perforated by the carotid canal. Posteriorly the mastoid part articulates with the parietal and occipital bones and contains air cells that develop only after birth. This part of the temporal bone also houses the stylomastoid foramen, which lies posterior to the styloid process and transmits the facial nerve. The fourth part of the temporal bone (the tympanic part) forms part of the wall of the external auditory meatus.

16.4 Maxilla

a. The maxilla is wholly a membranous bone
b. It articulates superiorly with the zygomatic and frontal bones
c. The roof of the maxillary sinus forms the orbital floor
d. The maxilla forms part of the nasolacrimal canal
e. It contains the greater palatine canal

71

The maxilla is wholly a membranous bone and plays an important part of the formation of the orbital floor, the lateral wall of the nose and the hard palate. It articulates superiorly with the lacrimal, nasal, zygomatic, and frontal bones. The pyramidal maxillary sinus dominates the bone, extending from its apex in the zygomatic process to its floor in the alveolar process. The sinus is an important inferior relation of the orbit, and its roof is grooved by the infraorbital canal. The sinus drains into the middle meatus via the hiatus semilunaris in its nasal wall. Lying just posterior to this hiatus is the greater palatine groove, which (by virtue of its articulation with the palatine bone) forms the greater palatine canal. The walls of the nasolacrimal duct are formed from the maxilla, lacrimal bone, and the inferior nasal concha.

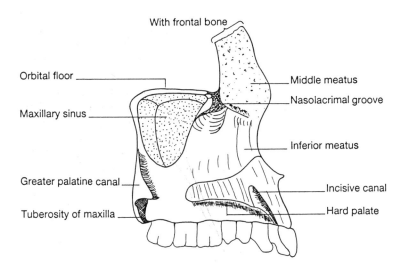

Fig 34 Medial view of the left maxilla

16.5 *Relations of the middle cranial fossa foramina*

a. The foramen spinosum connects the middle cranial and infratemporal fossae
b. The foramen ovale transmits the mandibular division of the trigeminal nerve
c. The foramen ovale transmits the middle meningeal artery
d. The internal carotid artery passes through the foramen lacerum
e. The deep petrosal nerve leaves the fossa via the pterygoid canal

Numerous foramina connect the middle cranial fossa with a number of extracranial sites. The foramen ovale, and the smaller foramen spinosum connect the middle cranial fossa with the infratemporal fossa. The middle meningeal artery (a terminal branch of the maxillary artery) passes through the foramen spinosum, whereas the foramen *o*vale transmits the mandibular division of the trigeminal nerve (*v*), the *a*ccessory meningeal artery, the *l*esser petrosal nerve and an *e*missary vein (OVALE). The foramen lacerum, which lies in the medial aspect of the middle cranial fossa, does not transmit any structures but the internal carotid artery passes across it. The deep petrosal nerve, containing sympathetic fibres bound for the pterygopalatine ganglion, leaves the fossa in conjunction with the greater petrosal nerve via the pterygoid canal.

16.6 *Foramina and fissures*

a. The jugular foramen transmits the ninth, tenth, and eleventh cranial nerves
b. The foramen magnum transmits the cranial part of the accessory nerve
c. The stylomastoid foramen transmits the facial nerve
d. The squamotympanic fissure transmits the chorda tympani
e. The hypoglossal canal passes through the bases of the occipital condyles

73

The jugular foramen (situated in the posterior cranial fossa) transmits the ninth, tenth, and eleventh cranial nerves, and the internal jugular vein. The accessory nerve consists of two parts: cranial, and spinal (which enters the skull via the foramen magnum). The stylomastoid foramen in the temporal bone transmits the facial nerve but the chorda tympani (a branch of the nervus intermedius that accompanies the facial nerve in the middle ear) does not exit via this foramen—it enters the infratemporal fossa via the petrotympanic fissure. The hypoglossal canal, which transmits the twelfth cranial nerve, transects the bases of the occipital condyles.

17: Gross anatomy of the head and neck

17.1 *Cervical vertebrae*

A typical cervical vertebra is characterised by:
a. A foramen transversarium
b. A circular shaped vertebral canal
c. A bifid spinal process
d. Large transverse processes
e. Kidney shaped body

There are seven cervical vertebrae: the atlas and axis (C1 and C2) are atypical and C7 has certain peculiar characteristics, so there are only four typical vertebrae (C3–C6). The foramen transversarium is found in the tranverse processes of all cervical vertebrae. Features characteristic of C3–C6 include a triangular shaped vertebral canal, bifid spinal processes, kidney shaped body, and small transverse processes. Occasionally the transverse process of C7 may be enlarged to form a cervical rib.

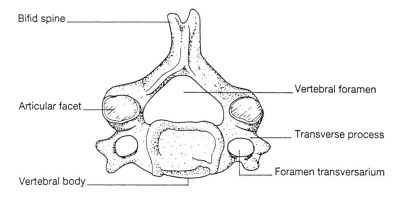

Fig 35 A typical cervical vertebra

17.2 *Cervical plexus*

a. The sensory roots emerge at the anterior border of the sternocleidomastoid
b. There is no C1 dermatome
c. The greater auricular nerve supplies the skin over the parotid gland
d. The ansa cervicalis is the motor supply to the strap muscles
e. The phrenic nerve root value is C3,4

The cervical plexus is formed by the anterior rami of the upper four cervical nerves after each has received a grey ramus from the superior cervical ganglion. It is covered by prevertebral fascia and its sensory roots pierce this before emerging at the posterior border of the sternocleidomastoid. There is no C1 dermatome but a loop from C1 passes to the hypoglossal nerve, from which fibres are transmitted to the superior root of the ansa cervicalis. The ansa cervicalis is the motor supply to the strap muscles and comprises the superior root (as described above) and an inferior root formed by the union of branches from C2 and C3. The greater auricular nerve (whose root value is C2,3) supplies the skin over the parotid gland, the angle of the mandible, and both sides of the ear lobe. The phrenic nerve is formed mainly from C4 fibres but also has contributions from C3 and C5. It is the sole motor supply to the diaphragm and its sensory fibres innervate the central dome of the diaphragm, the fibrous pericardium, part of the parietal pleura, and the diaphragmatic peritoneum.

17.3 *Carotid arteries*

a. The right common carotid arises from the aortic arch
b. The common carotid bifurcates at the level of the superior border of the thyroid cartilage
c. The internal carotid has no branches in the neck
d. The facial and lingual arteries are anterior branches of the external carotid
e. The external carotid divides into superficial temporal and maxillary branches before entering the parotid gland

The left common carotid artery is the third branch arising from the aortic arch; the right common carotid artery arises in the root of the neck from the brachiocephalic artery. The common carotid arteries bifurcate at the level of the superior border of the thyroid cartilage (C3), this bifurcation being marked by a distension of the artery known as the carotid sinus. The internal carotid artery has no branches in the neck. The branches of the external carotid artery may be described according to their origins: the ascending pharyngeal branch is the only one to arise from the medial aspect of the artery; superior thyroid, facial, and lingual arteries arise from the anterior aspect; the posterior auricular and occipital branches arise from the posterior aspect. The external carotid enters the parotid gland before dividing into its two terminal branches—the superficial temporal and maxillary arteries.

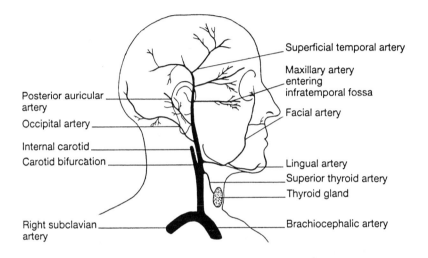

Fig 36 Right external carotid and its branches

17.4 *Relations of the carotid sheath*

a. The internal jugular vein lies medial to the carotid artery
b. The vagus nerve lies medial to the common carotid artery
c. The ansa cervicalis is embedded in the anterior wall of the sheath
d. The hypoglossal nerve lies superficial to the sheath
e. The sympathetic chain lies deep to the carotid sheath

The carotid sheath is made of a dense "feltwork" of areolar tissue surrounding the carotid arteries (both common and internal), the internal jugular vein, and the vagus nerve. The internal jugular vein has a lateral position in the sheath, whose wall is thinned over the vein to allow for dilation during increased blood flow. The vagus nerve is sandwiched between the common carotid medially and the internal jugular vein laterally. Other important neuronal relations of the sheath include the ansa cervicalis (which is embedded in the anterior wall), the sympathetic chain (which lies deep to the sheath), and the hypoglossal nerve (which passes anteriorly, lying superficial to the sheath).

17.5 *Structure and relations of the thyroid gland*

a. The gland may be connected to the tongue
b. The isthmus of the thyroid lies level with the second to fourth tracheal rings
c. The recurrent laryngeal nerve lies beside the superior thyroid artery
d. The external laryngeal nerve lies beside the inferior thyroid artery
e. The thyroid gland is enclosed by pretracheal fascia

The thyroid gland consists of two symmetrical lobes that are united in front of the second, third, and fourth tracheal rings by an isthmus of gland tissue. The thyroid gland develops in the floor of the primitive pharynx and descends to its adult position. The thyroglossal duct is a simple downgrowth that originates from the foramen caecum of the tongue. It passes ventrally between the first and second pharyngeal arches then caudally in front of the remaining arches to the commencement of the trachea. Remnants of the thyroglossal duct may produce cysts anywhere along the course of the duct. During thyroid surgery the two important relations that should be remembered are that of the recurrent laryngeal nerve (which is intimately related to the inferior thyroid artery), and the external laryngeal nerve (which runs with the superior thyroid artery). The entire, thyroid gland is enclosed by pretracheal fascia.

17.6 *Blood supply, venous and lymphatic drainage of the thyroid gland*

a. The superior thyroid artery arises from the external carotid artery
b. The inferior thyroid artery arises directly from the subclavian artery
c. The thyroid gland is drained by veins corresponding to its arteries
d. The inferior thyroid vein drains into the internal jugular vein
e. The thyroidea ima artery is present in 3% of individuals

The arterial supply to the thyroid gland is via the superior thyroid artery, arising from the anterior aspect of the external carotid and from the inferior thyroid artery (a branch of the thyrocervical trunk that arises from the first part of the subclavian artery). The thyroidea ima artery, which arises from the brachiocephalic trunk or directly from the arch of the aorta, enters the lower part of the isthmus in 3% of individuals. Drainage is via three veins: the superior thyroid (entering either the internal jugular or the facial vein); the middle thyroid (that passes directly into the internal jugular); the inferior thyroid veins (which form a plexus that drains the isthmus and lower poles into the left brachiocephalic vein).

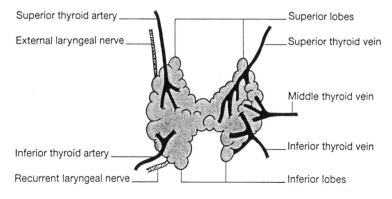

Superior thyroid artery — Superior lobes
External laryngeal nerve — Superior thyroid vein
Middle thyroid vein
Inferior thyroid artery — Inferior thyroid vein
Recurrent laryngeal nerve — Inferior lobes

Fig 37 Blood supply and venous drainage of the thyroid gland

17.7 Structure and relations of the submandibular gland

> a. The submandibular gland is a mixed mucous and serous gland
> b. It lies mainly deep to the mylohyoid
> c. It is crossed by the lingual artery
> d. This gland receives parasympathetic fibres from the chorda tympani
> e. The submandibular duct passes between the mylohyoid and the hyoglossus

The submandibular gland is a mixed mucous and serous gland consisting of a large superficial and a smaller deeper part that are continuous around the posterior border of the mylohyoid. The submandibular duct emerges from the superficial part of the gland and runs forward between the mylohyoid and the hyoglossus. It opens into the floor of the mouth beside the frenulum. An important anterior relation of the submandibular gland is the facial artery, which often grooves its surface. Parasympathetic secretomotor fibres originate in the chorda tympani, join the lingual nerve and synapse in the submandibular ganglion. Postganglionic fibres connect directly with the gland.

17.8 Relations of the parotid gland

> a. The parotid is predominantly a mucous gland
> b. The facial nerve divides in the superficial gland
> c. The retromandibular vein is the deepest structure of the parotid gland
> d. The parotid duct opens opposite the neck of the second upper molar tooth
> e. Parasympathetic fibres from the otic ganglion travel in the auriculotemporal nerve to the parotid gland

The parotid gland is predominantly a serous salivary gland surrounded by a tough capsule derived from the investing layer of deep cervical fascia. It is situated in the gap between the mastoid process and the sternomastoid, the ramus of the mandible and the styloid process. The parotid has a number of important relations. These are (from superficial to deep): the facial nerve (which divides into its terminal branches within the gland); the retromandibular vein (formed by the maxillary and superficial temporal veins and lies just deep to the facial nerve—by following its tributaries the surgeon is often able to identify the terminal branches of the facial nerve); the external carotid artery and its terminal branches (the superficial temporal and maxillary arteries) are the deepest structures in the gland (along with the auriculotemporal nerve, which carries postganglionic parasympathetic fibres from the otic ganglion). The parotid duct emerges from the anterior surface of the gland and pierces the buccinator before opening opposite the neck of the second upper molar tooth.

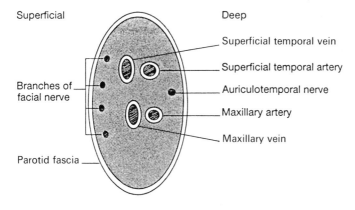

Fig 38 Horizontal cross section of the parotid gland

17.9 *Nervus intermedius*

a. The nervus intermedius enters the internal acoustic meatus with the facial nerve
b. Parasympathetic fibres synapse in its geniculate ganglion
c. The nervus intermedius provides secretomotor fibres to both the submandibular and the sublingual glands
d. The lesser petrosal nerve is derived from the nervus intermedius
e. The chorda tympani supplies taste to the anterior third of the tongue

The nervus intermedius contains secretomotor fibres arising from the superior salivatory nucleus, and sensory fibres which terminate in the nucleus of the solitary tract. It leaves the brain stem in conjunction with the facial nerve and enters the internal acoustic meatus. The geniculate ganglion, which marks a right angle bend in the nerve as it passes through the middle ear, is a sensory, not a parasympathetic, ganglion (similar to the dorsal root ganglions of the spinal cord). The chorda tympani, which arises from the nervus intermedius in the middle ear, carries secretomotor fibres that synapse in the submandibular ganglion before supplying the sublingual and submandibular glands. It also contains special sensory fibres that supply taste to the anterior two thirds of the tongue. The nervus intermedius gives off the greater petrosal nerve at the level of the geniculate ganglion. This nerve contains parasympathetic fibres that will synapse in the pterygopalatine ganglion before supplying the lacrimal gland.

17.10 *Facial muscles and their innervation*

a. Frontalis is supplied by the temporal branch of the seventh cranial nerve
b. Temporalis is supplied by the mandibular branch of the fifth cranial nerve
c. The anterior belly of digastric is supplied by the seventh cranial nerve
d. Buccinator is supplied by the buccal branch of the fifth cranial nerve
e. Platysma is supplied by the cervical branch of the seventh cranial nerve

A simple knowledge of embryology is useful when considering the innervation of the facial muscles. Those muscles derived from the first pharyngeal arch are the muscles of mastication and are supplied by branches of the mandibular division of the trigeminal nerve. Those derived from the second pharyngeal arch are used for facial expression, and are supplied by branches of the facial nerve. Temporalis, masseter and pterygoid are therefore all supplied by the trigeminal nerve, whereas frontalis, orbicularis oculi and oris, and platysma are supplied by the facial nerve. Buccinator is the exception, for while it plays a role in mastication by preventing food from accumulating in the cheek, it is derived from the second pharyngeal arch and is therefore supplied by the facial nerve. The digastric is derived from both the first and second arches; thus its anterior belly is supplied by the trigeminal nerve and its posterior belly by the facial nerve.

17.11 *Infratemporal fossa*

a. The medial boundary of the infratemporal fossa is the medial pterygoid plate
b. The mandibular nerve enters via the foramen ovale
c. The maxillary artery exits via the pterygomaxillary fissure
d. The middle meningeal artery exits via the foramen spinosum
e. The chorda tympani supplies secretomotor fibres to the otic ganglion in the fossa

The infratemporal fossa is a box like fossa situated behind the maxilla, below and behind the zygomatic arch. Its roof is formed by the greater wing of the sphenoid bone and by part of the squamous part of the temporal bone. The medial wall of the fossa is formed by the lateral pterygoid plate, the anterior wall by the maxilla, the posterior wall by the styloid apparatus, and the lateral wall by the mandibular ramus. The major vessel in the fossa is the maxillary artery and its largest tributary, the middle meningeal artery, exits via the foramen spinosum. The maxillary artery itself leaves the fossa through the pterygomaxillary fissure and so enters the pterygopalatine fossa. The mandibular division of the trigeminal nerve enters the fossa via the foramen ovale; this is the only branch of the trigeminal nerve that contains motor fibres. The otic ganglion, which is situated in the infratemporal fossa, receives preganglionic parasympathetic fibres from the lesser petrosal nerve.

Answers

1.1	d	**2.4**	b, d, e	**4.1**	a, b, d
1.2	a, c, d	**2.5**	c, d	**4.2**	a, b, d, e
1.3	b, d	**2.6**	a, b, c, e	**4.3**	a, c, e
1.4	c, e				
1.5	a, b, c, e	**3.1**	a, b, d	**5.1**	d
		3.2	a, b, c	**5.2**	b, c, d
2.1	c, d	**3.3**	c, d, e	**5.3**	b, c, e
2.2	a, b	**3.4**	a, d, e	**5.4**	a, b, e
2.3	a, c, d	**3.5**	a, b, c, e	**5.5**	a

5.6	a, b, c, d	**10.4**	a, d	**14.3**	a, d, e
5.7	a, c, e	**10.5**	a, c	**14.4**	a, c, d
5.8	a, b, c, e	**10.6**	a, b	**14.5**	b, d, e
		10.7	a, b, d		
6.1	a, b, c	**10.8**	a, e	**15.1**	a, b, e
6.2	a, c, e	**10.9**	b, c, d	**15.2**	a, c, d, e
6.3	a, d			**15.3**	b, d, e
6.4	b, c, e	**11.1**	d, e	**15.4**	a, c, d, e
		11.2	b, c, e	**15.5**	a, b, c
7.1	a, c, e	**11.3**	b, c, d	**15.6**	a, b, c
7.2	a, c, d	**11.4**	a, b, d		
7.3	a, b, c, e	**11.5**	c, d, e	**16.1**	a, b, e
7.4	b	**11.6**	a, b, e	**16.2**	b, c, e
7.5	b, e	**11.7**	b, c, d	**16.3**	a, b, c
7.6	a, b, d, e	**11.8**	a, d, e	**16.4**	a, b, c, d
				16.5	a, b, e
8.1	a, d, e	**12.1**	a, b, d, e	**16.6**	a, c, e
8.2	d, e	**12.2**	b, c, e		
8.3	a, c, e	**12.3**	a, c, e	**17.1**	a, c, e
		12.4	d, e	**17.2**	b, c, d
9.1	a, b, c			**17.3**	b, c, d
9.2	a, b, d, e	**13.1**	b, d, e	**17.4**	c, d, e
9.3	a, b, c	**13.2**	a, b, e	**17.5**	a, b, e
9.4	b, c, e	**13.3**	a, b, c, d	**17.6**	a, e
9.5	a, d	**13.4**	c, d, e	**17.7**	a, d, e
		13.5	a, b, d, e	**17.8**	b, d, e
10.1	b, c, e			**17.9**	a, c
10.2	a, b, d, e	**14.1**	a, b, d, e	**17.10**	a, b, e
10.3	a, b, e	**14.2**	a, b, e	**17.11**	b, c, d

Microbiology

1: General microbiology

1.1 General characteristics of bacteria

a. Bacteria are prokaryotic cells
b. The cells contain DNA and RNA
c. The nuclear DNA is enclosed in a membrane
d. Bacteria possess intracellular organelles
e. They reproduce by binary fission

Bacteria are prokaryotic cells that contain DNA and RNA. The nuclear DNA is not enclosed in a membrane but lies free in the cytoplasm, which is devoid of intracellular organelles. Reproduction is by binary fission.

1.2 Bacterial structure

a. Porous cell walls make up to 20% of dry weight
b. Cell membranes provide an osmotic barrier
c. Plasmids contain RNA fragments
d. Mesosomes are found in the cytoplasm
e. Flagella and pili are responsible for motility

Most bacteria (except L-forms and mycoplasmas) have a cell wall that makes up approximately 10–20% of the dry weight. All walls contain a mucocomplex containing muramic acid and are porous to all but very large molecules. The cell membrane, unlike the inert cell wall, is an important osmotic barrier and the site of a number of important enzymes. Mesosomes are cytoplasmic sacs with intense enzymic activity associated with division septa. Plasmids contain DNA fragments and may be responsible for conferring antibiotic resistance. Flagella (made of long fibrillary proteins) are responsible for motility; pili are associated with conjugation.

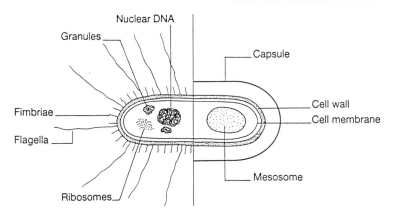

Fig 39 Bacterial structure

1.3 *Metabolism and growth*

a. Heterotrophs are able to synthesise all their organic requirements
b. All bacteria need CO_2 to initiate growth
c. Respiration and fermentation are two forms of oxidation
d. Aerobic bacteria may employ fermentation
e. Strict anaerobes rely entirely on respiration for energy

Autotrophs are able to utilise simple inorganic compounds but heterotrophs cannot synthesise all their organic requirements. All bacteria need CO_2 to initiate growth; usually a trace is enough but a few species need 3–5% in the atmosphere. Energy comes mainly from oxidation, the two forms of which are: (1) respiration (usually dependent upon cytochrome with CO_2 and H_2O as end products); and (2) fermentation (hydrogen is transferred to an organic compound with pyruvic or lactic end products). Aerobic bacteria obtain energy mainly by respiration, though most also employ fermentation (these are termed facultative anaerobes). Strict anaerobes rely entirely on fermentation for energy production.

1.4 *Culture of bacteria*

> a. Nutrient broth should be sterilised by heat and have a pH of 7.3
> b. Blood agar consists of nutrient agar and defibrinated horse blood
> c. Reducing agents support the growth of aerobes
> d. Desoxycholate–citrate agar is a "selective medium"
> e. MacConkey agar distinguishes between lactose and non-lactose fermenting microorganisms

Most bacteria will grow in an artificial medium resembling their normal habitat. Nutrient broth is a watery extract of meat, containing partly digested protein, carbohydrate, and electrolytes. It is sterilised by heat and has a pH of 7.3. Blood agar consists of nutrient agar with added defibrinated horse blood and is a good medium for fastidious and delicate bacteria. Strict anaerobes require reducing agents (such as sodium thioglycollate, minced cooked meat or metallic iron) to support their growth. Selective media contain chemicals that inhibit the growth of some bacteria only (for example desoxycholate–citrate agar, which permits the growth of salmonellae but inhibits *Escherichia coli*). MacConkey agar (which contains lactose) is a differential medium that distinguishes between lactose and non-lactose fermenting microorganisms.

1.5 *Gram staining*

> The Gram stain involves:
> a. Application of gentian violet
> b. Application of Lugol's iodine
> c. Application of strong carbol fuchsin
> d. Treatment with acetone
> e. Counterstaining with methylene blue

The sequential application of gentian violet and Lugol's iodine results in the deposition of a black–purple complex in the bacteria. After treatment with acetone some types of bacteria retain the complex and remain darkly stained (Gram positive), while others lose the complex and become colourless (Gram negative). The latter are usually stained pink for contrast using dilute carbol fuchsin. Methylene blue is the counterstain used when producing a Ziehl–Neelsen stain for acid fast bacilli.

1.6 *Microbacterial pathogenicity*

Invasiveness is enhanced by:
a. Adherence of microorganisms
b. Local tissue damage
c. Hyaluronidase
d. Coagulase
e. Haemolysins

The virulence of a pathogen depends on its invasiveness (its ability to enter the host, multiply, and spread) and its toxigenicity; these are largely independent characteristics. Invasiveness will be enhanced by the ability of the microorganism to adhere to target cells and by local tissue damage. Spread of the microorganism will be aided by hyaluronidase (which dissolves collagen); coagulases will precipitate fibrin clots, so walling off the bacteria from host defences; haemolysins will aid invasiveness by killing host phagocytes.

1.7 *Toxins*

a. Exotoxins are proteins
b. Endotoxins are present in all Gram negative bacteria
c. Both endotoxins and exotoxins are heat stable
d. Endotoxins have a specific pharmacological action
e. Exotoxins have greater potency than endotoxins

Traditionally toxins fall into two categories (exotoxins and endotoxins) although the distinction is not absolutely clear. Exotoxins are proteins (mostly enzymes), endotoxins are made from the lipopolysaccharide components of the bacterial cell wall. All Gram negative bacteria (such as salmonella, coliforms, and neisseria) contain similar endotoxins whether they are pathogens or not. Exotoxins are heat labile, strongly antigenic and are generally much more potent than endotoxins. They also have a specific pharmacological action, unlike endotoxins which have a non-specific acute inflammatory action.

1.8 *Physical methods of sterilisation and disinfection*

a. Ultraviolet radiation causes disinfection
b. Gamma radiation is used to sterilise syringes
c. Pasteurisation kills all vegetative organisms
d. Sterilisation is produced by dry heat at 100°C for 1 hour
e. Sterilisation is reduced by steam at 100°C for 1 hour at a pressure of 30 psi

Sterilisation means the destruction or removal of *all* micro-organisms and is an absolute term whereas disinfection means the destruction or removal of *most* microorganisms. Ultraviolet radiation is strongly absorbed by proteins and nucleic acids so producing genetic mutations, enzyme inactivation, and death. It is a commonly used disinfectant in laboratory cabinets. Gamma radiation (for example, using ^{60}Co) is frequently employed in industry for sterilising prepacked plastic syringes, et cetera. Pasteurisation involves temperatures of 80°C for 10 minutes at half an atmosphere of pressure. Steam generated at this pressure and temperature by this procedure will kill vegetative organisms but will not kill spores; pasteurisation is therefore a method of disinfection. Sterilisation by dry heat requires temperatures of 160°C for 1 hour. Using an autoclave to generate moist heat under pressure (134°C for 3 minutes at 30 psi) will kill all organisms, including resistant spores.

1.9 *Normal flora of the eye*

> a. *Staphylococcus epidermidis* is the most common organism inhabiting the eye
> b. *Staphylococcus aureus* is a normal flora
> c. *Propionibacterium granulosum* is the most common anaerobe
> d. *Demodex follicularum* is a yeast found on the eye lashes
> c. There are no viruses existing as normal eye flora

The commensal organisms present on the body surface are known as the normal flora. These are mostly saprophytes that live harmlessly on the skin and mucous membranes without invading or causing disease except in exceptional circumstances or when outside their normal habitat. The eye is sterile in utero but acquires normal flora during birth. *Staphylococcus epidermidis* is found in up to 70% of eyes, and *Staphylococcus aureus* in approximately 45%. The most common anaerobe is *Propionibacterium acnes*, which has been implicated in some forms of chronic endophthalmitis and blepharitis. Protozoan commensals include *Demodex follicularum* (found on the eye lashes in almost everyone over 70 years of age). Up to 100 fungi (including *Pityrosporon orbiculari*, a yeast found on the lashes and lid margins) have been found to normally inhabit the eye. There are no viral commensals of the eye.

2: Cocci

2.1 *General properties of staphylococci*

> a. Staphylococci are Gram positive bacteria
> b. They are aerobic and facultatively anaerobic
> c. Staphylococci are catalase negative
> d. *Staphylococcus epidermidis* is coagulase positive
> e. These organisms grow on simple media

Staphylococci are Gram positive cocci that grow in clusters like bunches of grapes on simple media. They are aerobic, facultatively anaerobic and are distinguished from streptococci in that they produce catalase. The pathogenic *Staphylococcus aureus* may be distinguished from the usually non-pathogenic *Staphylococcus epidermidis* by virtue of its coagulase activity.

2.2 *Staphylococcus aureus*

This organism:
a. Contains lysozyme
b. Has poor adherence
c. Produces entero and epidermolytic toxins
d. Has an opsonisation resistant capsule
e. Contains protein A

Staphylococcus aureus is carried on the skin of many normal people (especially in the anterior nares) and infection may often be endogenous. Strains may spread from carriers (such as those with septic lesions) via the air, by direct, and (most importantly) by indirect contact. The pathogenicity of *Staph. aureus* is enhanced by a number of factors that include lysozymes, coagulase and hyaluronidase. It also adheres well to cell surfaces, has an opsonisation resistant capsule, and produces a protein A that is thought to decrease phagocytosis and inhibit complement activation. Toxins produced by this organism include an epidermolytic toxin (responsible for the "scalded skin" syndrome), and an enterotoxin that causes food poisoning.

2.3 *Streptococci*

a. Streptococci are common ocular pathogens
b. They are Gram positive and catalase positive
c. *Streptococcus pyogenes* is a β haemolytic streptococcus Lancefield group A
d. *Streptococcus pneumoniae* is an α haemolytic diplococcus
e. *Streptococcus pyogenes* produces an erythrogenic toxin

Streptococci are Gram positive cocci that are catalase negative and are uncommon ocular pathogens. *Streptococcus pyogenes* (which causes over 90% of streptococcal infections in humans) is a β haemolytic streptococcus Lancefield group A. It produces an erythrogenic toxin and is responsible for the generalised erythematous rash seen in scarlet fever. *Streptococcus pneumoniae* is an α haemolytic diplococcus, which may occasionally cause meningitis as well as pneumonia.

2.4 *Neisseriae*

a. These are aerobic Gram positive cocci
b. They grow on simple media
c. The gonococcus contains IgA proteases
d. The meningococcus is a normal flora of the nasopharynx
e. Silver nitrate inhibits growth of the gonococcus

The genus *Neisseria* comprises two important pathogens, *Neisseria meningitides* (meningococcus) and *Neisseria gonorrhoea* (gonococcus). They are aerobic Gram negative cocci that require special media such as heated blood agar with an increased carbon dioxide concentration to grow. Both have endotoxin type activity and possess IgA proteases that cleave immunoglobulins. The meningococcus is a strict parasite that colonises the human nasopharynx, and dies rapidly outside the body. The gonococcus is responsible for ophthalmia neonatorum—in 1881 Credé reduced the incidence of this condition from 10% to 0.3% by applying silver nitrate to the eyes of neonates.

3: Bacilli

3.1 *General properties of mycobacteria*

a. These are aerobic non-sporing rods
b. They stain with a Ziehl–Neelsen stain
c. Mycobacteria grow on simple media
d. They have a generation time of 12–24 hours
e. All species are pathogenic to humans

Mycobacteria are aerobic non-sporing rods with waxy cell walls which prevent them taking up Gram stain. However, they stain with hot strong carbol fuchsin (Ziehl–Neelsen stain), which is retained despite attempts to remove it with mineral acids and alcohol (that is, they are acid and alcohol fast bacilli). They will grow only on enriched media such as Löwenstein–Jensen medium (which contains egg). They also have a very slow generation time of 12–24 hours, which means that cultures may take up to 8 weeks to grow. Mycobacteria are widely distributed in nature but only a few species are pathogenic to humans.

3.2 *Mycobacterium tuberculosis*

a. The primary host of this organism is the human
b. It produces an endotoxin
c. It is resistant to intracellular enzymes
d. *Mycobacterium tuberculosis* produces a non-caseating granuloma
e. Prophylaxis is by a live attenuated vaccine

Mycobacterium tuberculosis is never a commensal organism: the human is its primary host. It does not produce a toxin nor does it inhibit phagocytosis (its pathogenicity depends on its ability to resist destruction by intracellular enzymes). The characteristic lesion caused by this organism is a caseating granuloma made up of macrophages and macrophage derived cells. Prophylaxis is attained using the live attenuated bovine strain known as the bacille Calmette–Guérin (BCG).

3.3 *Sporing bacteria*

a. Spores consist of a cortex with concentric protective layers
b. Most of these organisms are Gram positive bacilli
c. Spores are a means of reproduction
d. Spores are metabolically active
e. Spores are resistant to heat, radiation and chemicals

Characteristically spores consist of a central cortex surrounded by a layered outer coat made from laminated keratin, that is in turn surrounded by a loose endospore. Nearly all are produced by Gram positive bacilli that are predominantly saprophytes but include some potent human pathogens. Spores are not a means of reproduction, nor are they metabolically active—they are a resting and defensive form of existence. Sporulation allows the organism to survive for long periods as spores are extraordinarily resistant to heat, radiation, desiccation, and chemicals.

3.4 *Bacilli*

a. Spores are visible as refractile bodies
b. *Bacillus anthracis* is non-motile and non-haemolytic
c. *Bacillus anthracis* is encapsulated
d. *Bacillus cereus* produces a lethal toxin
e. Some bacilli produce antibiotics

Members of the genus *Bacillus* are aerobic Gram positive rods whose spores are visible as colourless refractile bodies. *Bacillus anthracis* causes anthrax and is an encapsulated organism capable of producing exotoxins. *Bacillus cereus* produces a lethal toxin and causes food poisoning in humans. *Bacillus brevis* can produce bacitracin—a potent antibiotic.

3.5 *General properties of clostridia*

These organisms:
a. Are facultative anaerobes
b. Live in soil water and decaying vegetation
c. Swarm on solid media
d. Produce potent endotoxins
e. May have a saprophytic relationship with humans

Clostridia are large Gram positive rods and, being obligate anaerobes, will grow only in anaerobic jars or in the presence of a reducing agent. The clostridia comprise many saprophytes living in soil water and decaying vegetation and are found in the gut of humans and other animals. Some produce powerful exotoxins, and they act as potent pathogens if introduced into human tissues.

3.6 *Clostridium tetani and Clostridium perfringens*

a. *Clostridium tetani* has drumstick spores
b. Both cause local damage to tissues
c. Produce neurotoxins and enterotoxins respectively
d. The Nagler reaction distinguishes between the two in culture
e. Are both sensitive to penicillin

Clostridium tetani is the causative organism of tetanus and produces large spherical terminal spores which have a drumstick appearance. *Clostridium perfringens* is the most common cause of gas gangrene and forms large haemolytic colonies on blood agar. Each disease will develop only if the organism is implanted into the tissues by deep penetrating injuries, but only *C. perfringens* will bring about local damage to the tissues by its powerful exotoxins. Tetanus toxin is a specific exotoxin that affects the presynaptic terminals of inhibitory interneurones, causing the characteristic tonic spasm of the voluntary muscles. Some strains of *C. perfringens* will produce an enterotoxin that causes food poisoning. The Nagler reaction is an identification technique used to distinguish different types of *C. perfringens*. Both organisms are sensitive to penicillin.

3.7 *Gram positive bacilli*

a. *Corynebacterium diphtheriae* produces a powerful exotoxin
b. *Listeria monocytogenes* is an extracellular parasite
c. *Bacillus cereus* is the most common ocular pathogen
d. *Nocardia asteroides* produces no toxins
e. Are prevalent in humoral immune deficiencies

Gram positive aerobic bacilli are rare causes of ocular infections but may have a devastating effect on the eye. *Corynebacterium diphtheriae* produces a powerful exotoxin that prevents ribosomes from incorporating amino acids into peptide chains, but it is only pathogenic if the infection is intraocular. *Listeria monocytogenes* is an invasive intracellular parasite which adheres well to the conjunctival epithelium. *Nocardia asteroides* is an opportunistic intracellular parasite that produces no toxins or virulence factors and is responsible for some chorioretinal and iris lesions. The anaerobic *Bacillus cereus* is the most common ocular pathogen in this group, and is responsible for 25% of endophthalmitis following penetrating ocular trauma. All the above are more prevalent in cell-mediated immune deficiencies than humoral deficiencies.

3.8 *Enterobacteriaceae*

a. All are oxidase negative and produce endotoxins
b. *Escherichia coli* are lactose fermenting and non-motile organisms
c. Klebsiella are urease negative and lactose fermenting
d. Salmonellae are enteric commensals
e. Proteus is urease positive

The enterobacteriaceae are intestinal Gram negative bacilli, most of which are commensals in the gastrointestinal tract that may become pathogenic in other sites such as the urinary tract and wounds. All are oxidase negative and produce endotoxins. *Escherichia coli* are lactose fermenting urease negative organisms and are usually motile; all are commensals apart from the occasional enteropathogenic strain. Klebsiella are also urease negative and lactose fermenting gut commensals. Salmonella and proteus are both lactose-fermenting motile organisms: proteus is a urease positive gut commensal and salmonellae are urease negative enteric pathogens.

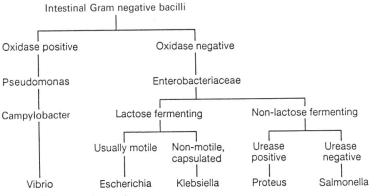

Fig 40 **The enterobacteriaceae**

97

3.9 *Gram negative bacilli*

These include:
a. *Moraxella lacunata*
b. Koch–Weeks bacillus
c. *Brucella abortus*
d. *Pasteurella multocida*
e. *Francisella tularensis*

Moraxella lacunata was first discovered by an ophthalmologist and is known to cause central corneal ulcers and blepharitis although the non-liquefaciens form is now more common. The Koch–Weeks bacillus (previously known as *Haemophilus aegyptius*) causes a form of conjunctivitis endemic in North Africa and the Gulf States of the USA. *Brucella abortus* is a highly pathogenic organism which may cause a nummular keratitis and uveitis. *Pasteurella multocida* is found in the saliva of dogs and humans and may cause virulent wound infections following bites. *Francisella tularensis* is another rare but highly pathogenic Gram negative rod.

3.10 *Pseudomonas aeruginosa*

a. This organism is facultatively anaerobic
b. Iron is essential for its growth
c. Pseudomonas is able to penetrate healthy corneal epithelium
d. It produces numerous proteases
e. It produces a "toxin A"

Pseudomonas aeruginosa is an oxidase positive, Gram negative, strictly aerobic bacterium. It is a virulent ocular pathogen. It appears to be dependent on iron for growth and changes in iron metabolism are thought to affect its virulence with respect to corneal infection. It does not penetrate healthy corneal epithelium well but the action of numerous proteases enables it to pass quickly through traumatised epithelium. It also produces a "toxin A" with a mechanism similar to that of diphtheria toxin, which breaks protein glycol matrices. Predisposing factors to pseudomonal infection include corneal trauma, thermal burns, vitamin A deficiency, and immune suppression.

3.11 *Anaerobic ocular pathogens*

These include:
a. *Propionibacterium acnes*
b. *Bacteroides fragilis*
c. *Clostridium perfringens*
d. *Escherichia coli*
e. *Actinomyces israeli*

Although *Propionibacterium acnes* is a normal commensal of the eye, it has been implicated in some cases of chronic endophthalmitis, phakoantigenic uveitis, and some forms of blepharitis. Bacteroides are strictly anaerobic Gram negative rods that are gut commensals and account for approximately 12% of anaerobic ocular infections. *Clostridium perfringens* may cause a conjunctivitis or necrotising keratitis that can on occasion progress to panophthalmitis with retinal necrosis. *Escherichia coli* is an aerobic organism. *Actinomyces israeli* is often implicated in lacrimal canalicular infections and is characterised by the presence of sulphur granules.

4: Chlamydia

4.1 *Chlamydia trachomatis*

a. These are obligate intracellular bacteria
b. All serotypes are glycogen positive
c. Serotypes D–K cause classic endemic trachoma
d. Lymphogranuloma venereum is caused by serotypes L1, 2 and 3
e. This organism causes psittacosis

Chlamydia are obligate intracellular bacteria that possess no cell wall. The genus includes *Chlamydia trachomatis*, *Chlamydia psittaci* and *Chlamydia pneumoniae*. *C. trachomatis* may be further divided into a number of serotypes by microimmune fluorescence tests: all are glycogen positive and have humans as their only host. Serotypes A, B and C cause classic endemic trachoma and serotypes D to K cause adult inclusion conjunctivitis (which is sexually transmitted). Subtypes L1, 2 and 3 cause lymphogranuloma venereum.

4.2 *Life cycle of Chlamydia trachomatis*

a. An elemental body attaches to and penetrates the cell wall
b. The elemental body is non-infectious
c. The initial body is the replicative form
d. Replication lasts for approximately 1 week
e. Different strains have different amino acid needs

Chlamydia trachomatis exists in two forms: the elemental body (the infectious form that attaches to a host cell); and the initial body (the replicative form). Once the elemental body penetrates the cell it is enclosed in a cytoplasmic vesicle that is spared lysosomal degradation and after 6–8 hours becomes organised into an initial body. The metabolically active form divides for approximately 24 hours before regressing to the elemental form. Different strains have been found to have different amino acid needs: serotypes A, B and C require tryptophan whereas L1, 2 and 3 need methionine.

4.3 *Laboratory diagnostic aids*

These include:
a. Giemsa staining of smears
b. Gram staining
c. ELISA
d. Antibody detection in serum and tears
e. Electron microscopy

The main laboratory aids to chlamydial identification are Giemsa staining of smears to identify inclusions, enzyme linked immunosorbent assay (ELISA) techniques, and detection of antibody to chlamydia in the serum and tears.

5: General virology

5.1 *General properties of viruses*

a. Virus particles are acellular
b. The capsid encloses the nucleic acid
c. All capsids are icosahedral in shape
d. The viral genome may contain both DNA and RNA
e. Viruses replicate by binary fission

Unlike fungi and bacteria, virus particles are acellular and therefore in order to replicate a virion must enter a cell to "borrow" its metabolism. The virion consists of the viral genome (either DNA or RNA) enclosed in a protein shell. This is composed of identical subunits (capsids), which are in turn composed of identical subunits (capsomers). Capsids may be icosahedral or helical in shape and are often surrounded by a lipoprotein envelope.

5.2 *Viral replication*

a. Adsorption is the first step
b. Penetration is solely by viropexis
c. The capsid is removed by host cell enzymes
d. Nucleic acid replication is the same for both DNA and RNA viruses
e. New virus particles are released by cell lysis

Viral replication has a number of stages. The first of these is adsorption—the virus particle becomes attached to a cell by random collision, by electrostatic attachment, or by specific host cell receptors. This is followed by penetration (by viropexis or by fusion of the viral envelope and cell membrane). The capsid is removed by host cell enzymes and nucleic acid replication (which differs for DNA and RNA viruses) takes place. Assembly of the new nucleic acid and protein capsid is followed by a period of maturation before the new virus particles are released by cell lysis or by budding through the cell membrane.

5.3 *Replication of nucleic acids*

a. All DNA viruses replicate in the nucleus of the host cell
b. Most DNA viruses use host cell polymerases
c. RNA viruses replicate in the host's cytoplasm
d. RNA viruses copy RNA from the host's RNA using host enzymes
e. Reverse transcriptase makes DNA from an RNA template

Nucleic acid replication differs between viruses. Most DNA viruses (except the poxviruses) replicate in the nucleus using host cell enzymes to make messenger RNA and to replicate DNA. Nucleic acid replication in RNA viruses occurs in the cytoplasm and may proceed in a number of ways. Unlike the DNA viruses, RNA viruses are unable to borrow host cell enzymes because none exist for copying RNA from RNA. One way that these organisms overcome this problem is to use a reverse transcriptase enzyme that can make DNA from an RNA template.

5.4 *Virus transmission*

> a. Cytomegalovirus and rubella are spread transplacentally
> b. Herpes simplex virus can be transmitted vertically
> c. Paramyxoviruses are transmitted by airborne routes
> d. Enteroviruses are acid and bile stable
> e. Herpes simplex virus may be transmitted horizontally

Transmission of viruses may be divided into two main categories: (1) vertical transmission, when a virus is passed from the mother to the offspring; (2) horizontal transmission, when a virus is passed from one individual to another after birth. Cytomegalovirus and rubella may be transmitted vertically via a transplacental route and so cause developmental abnormalities. The herpes simplex virus may be transmitted vertically (during birth) and horizontally by direct contact. Other forms of horizontal transmission include the faecal–oral route utilised by the enteroviruses (which tend to be acid and bile stable) and the airborne-respiratory route by the paramyxoviruses. Parenteral (through the skin) routes are important in hepatitis B and rabies.

5.5 *Results of virus infection*

> a. Formation of multinucleate cells
> b. Cell death
> c. Persistence, with virus in a non-replicative state
> d. Latency, which implies integration of viral DNA into the host DNA
> e. Malignant and teratogenic change

The cytopathic effect (CPE) is the visible effect of virus infection on the cell (for example, cell shrinking, cell rounding, and production of inclusions) in the formation of giant multinucleate cells. This may be followed by cell death, caused by cytolysis or inhibition of cell metabolism. Chronic infection may be in one of two forms: (1) persistence, in which the virus replicates at a low rate; (2) latency, where the virus does not replicate and the viral genome is integrated into the host DNA. The other sequela of virus infection is transformation—the virus confers on the cell new properties of growth and morphology (malignant and teratogenic change).

5.6 *Spread of viruses within the host*

> a. Spread may occur along body surfaces
> b. Herpes zoster has a retrograde neuronal spread
> c. Epstein–Barr virus is found in platelets
> d. Smallpox travels in monocytes
> e. Colorado tick virus is found in red blood cells

Viruses spread by numerous routes within the host, one of the most common being along body surfaces (used by the respiratory and enteric viruses). Systemic spread is often via neuronal routes—as in the case of herpes simplex and zoster viruses, which have a retrograde neuronal flow. Haematogenous spread is also common, with smallpox travelling in monocytes, Epstein–Barr virus in lymphocytes and Colorado tick virus in red blood cells.

5.7 *Virus serology and rapid diagnostic tests*

> a. The complement fixation test measures the reaction between viral antigen and a specific antibody
> b. In the complement fixation test indicator erythrocytes are lysed in a positive test
> c. Electron microscopy can identify viruses in tears
> d. Reverse passive haemagglutination is used in detection of hepatitis B surface antigens
> e. ELISA employs antibodies conjugated to radioisotopes

Virus isolation has been superseded by virus serology, and other rapid diagnostic methods in the management of viral infections. Complement fixation (reaction between viral antigen and a specific antibody, measured by the consumption of added complement) is the test most widely used. In a positive test the indicator erythrocytes are not lysed by the complement as it has already been consumed by the antigen/antibody reaction. Electron microscopy has been used to demonstrate viruses in faeces, vesicle fluids and tears but needs an electron dense stain to provide contrast. Reverse passive haemagglutination may be used to detect hepatitis B surface antigen. Enzyme linked immunosorbent assay (ELISA) and RIA (radioimmunoassay) are also useful diagnostic aids.

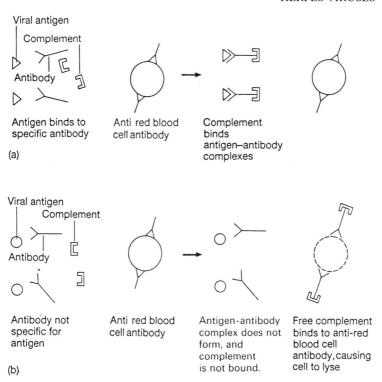

Fig 41 **The complement fixation test: (a) positive; (b) negative**

6: Herpes viruses

6.1 *Herpes viruses*

a. Are single stranded DNA viruses
b. Have a helical capsid
c. Exhibit latency
d. Include varicella zoster virus
e. Include the Epstein–Barr virus

The herpes viruses are double stranded DNA viruses that possess an icosahedral capsid. They include herpes simplex, varicella zoster, cytomegalovirus and the Epstein–Barr virus. After the primary infection some herpesviruses become latent in neuronal sites within the body and under certain conditions may reactivate causing renewed disease—latency of herpes simplex and varicella zoster viruses.

6.2 *Herpes simplex virus*

a. HSV-1 may cause acute gingivostomatitis
b. HSV-2 causes herpes gladiatorum
c. HSV-1 may become latent in the trigeminal ganglion
d. HSV-2 produces genital infections
e. Serology may be used to detect secondary infections

Herpes simplex viruses may be divided into two subtypes by clinical, biological and serological criteria. HSV-1 is associated mainly with oral infection and, although the primary infection in young children is often subclinical, it causes an acute gingivostomatitis in approximately 10% of cases. A rarer primary form of HSV-1 infection is herpes gladiatorum (scrumpox). HSV-1 may become latent in the trigeminal ganglion and may cause recurrent disease in response to a number of stimuli. HSV-2 is primarily an infection of young adults, in whom it causes a genital infection that may be accomplished by a mild meningitis. Diagnostic techniques such as ELISA and DNA probes are of use only in primary infections.

6.3 *Pathogenicity of HSV-1*

a. The viral envelope is highly immunogenic
b. The HSV genome can code for 10–15 proteins
c. The genome is the prime determinant of virulence
d. Stromal disease is caused by a replicating virus
e. The immune response determines the frequency of recurrence

The pathogenicity of the herpes simplex virus is increased in the immunosuppressed, in malignancy and by the application of topical steroids. The HSV genome can code for approximately 50–75 proteins and because of these different combinations each strain will produce a characteristic length, pattern and degree of invasion. The arrangement of the viral genome is thought to be the prime determinant of virulence in the non-immunosuppressed patient. The viral envelope is highly immunogenic and stromal disease is thought to be caused by a hypersensitivity reaction to viral antigen—not by replicating viruses. The genome is also the prime factor governing the frequency of recurrent disease.

6.4 *Latency of HSV-1*

a. The ganglion is the sole reservoir during latency
b. Latent viruses are phenotypically altered
c. Two or more virus strains may be present in one ganglion
d. Recurrence may be triggered by fever
e. Reactivated virus may spread to another ganglion

The ganglion is the sole reservoir of herpes simplex during latency. "Super infection" of the ganglion (that is, other strains of the virus cannot infect a ganglion when another strain is "in residence" even if this second strain is highly virulent) is not thought to occur. The latent virus is not phenotypically altered and reactivation may be triggered by fever, stress, ultraviolet light, menstruation, and trauma. Once reactivated the virus may spread to another ganglion and become latent once more.

6.5 *Varicella zoster virus*

a. Varicella zoster is the causative agent of chickenpox
b. It is spread by the respiratory route
c. Humoral immunity is essential in maintaining the virus in the latent state
d. Exposure to X rays can reactivate the virus
e. Shingles is most common in the thoracic region

Varicella zoster virus (VZV) is the causative agent of chicken-pox (characterised by successive crops of intraepidermal vesicles on the trunk, face and in the mouth). Chickenpox is highly infectious and is spread by the respiratory route. The virus may become latent in a number of ganglia, the most common sites being the trigeminal followed by the thoracic lumbar and cervical nerve ganglia. Cell mediated immunity is essential in maintaining the virus in the latent state. Reactivation, leading to shingles, may be caused by immunosuppression or X ray therapy.

6.6 *Cytomegalovirus*

a. Childhood infection is usually symptomatic
b. The virus may be spread vertically or horizontally
c. The virus is shed by 1% of all neonates
d. Cytomegalovirus may be shed from genital and urinary tracts
e. It becomes latent in lymphocytes

Cytomegalovirus infection is very common, but it is subclinical in 80% of cases. The virus may be shed from the genital and urinary tracts and becomes latent in lymphoctyes. The virus may be reactivated during pregnancy, and results in asymptomatic infection of the fetus; however, primary infection during pregnancy (especially in the first trimester) may cause fetal abnormalities. The virus is shed at birth by 1% of infants, with 10% of these having minor abnormalities such as hearing deficits and 2–3% exhibiting cytomegalic inclusion disease.

6.7 *Problems caused by cytomegalovirus*

a. Microphthalmia
b. Post transfusion mononucleosis
c. Childhood hepatitis
d. Retinitis in the immunocompetent patient
e. Transplant rejection

Congenital infection with cytomegalovirus may cause cytomegalic inclusion disease, which can produce strabismus, chorioretinitis and microphthalmia. It causes a number of problems for the immunocomprised individual including CMV retinitis (in AIDS patients) transplant rejection and CMV pneumonia. Post transfusion mononucleosis and childhood hepatitis are rare complications of infection with this organism.

7: Airborne and enteric viruses

7.1 *Measles*

a. Measles is caused by a paramyxovirus
b. Infection is often subclinical
c. Conjunctivitis is often a prodromal finding
d. The incidence of encephalitis is approximately 1 in 10 000
e. SSPE may be associated with chorioretinitis and maculopathy

Measles is caused by a paramyxovirus, infection being characterised by pyrexia, prodromal cough, coryza, and conjunctivitis. Subclinical infections do not occur. The most common complication is a secondary bacterial respiratory infection but encephalitis occurs in 1 in 1000 cases. Subacute sclerosing panencephalitis (SSPE) is a rare, slowly progressive and fatal encephalitis caused by slow viral infection—it has been associated with chorioretinitis and maculopathy.

7.2 *Rubella*

a. Rubella belongs to the togavirus family
b. Infection is subclinical in 80% of children
c. Vertical transmission is most dangerous in the second trimester
d. Recent infection is detected by a raised IgG titre
e. Immunisation is by a live attenuated vaccine

The rubella virus is spread by droplet infection. The disease is subclinical in 80% of small children and 10% of adults. Its importance lies in the increased probability of congenital abnormalities in children born to mothers infected during the first trimester of pregnancy. Recent infection is characterised by a raised IgM titre that will remain high for approximately 2 months after the initial infection (a raised IgG titre is an indication only of previous infection). A live attenuated vaccine is given to all children under the age of 12 years.

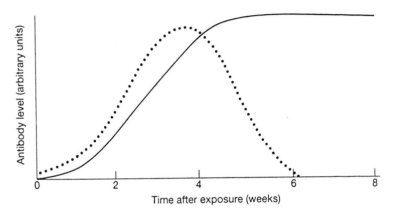

Fig 42 **Maternal antibody levels in rubella infection. (—) IgM; (•••) IgG**

7.3 Congenital abnormalities caused by rubella

a. Cataracts
b. A patent ductus arteriosus
c. Microphthalmia
d. Conductive deafness
e. Glaucoma

If a woman is infected with rubella during pregnancy the virus spreads to the placenta and hence to the fetus. Miscarriages or stillbirths are common sequelae to infection as are congenital defects such as cataracts, microphthalmia, glaucoma, nerve deafness, and congenital heart problems such as a patent ductus arteriosus.

7.4 *Mumps*

a. This disease is caused by a paramyxovirus
b. Rising antibody titres to V antigen indicates recent infection
c. Mumps may cause a dacryoadenitis
d. It may cause meningoencephalitis
e. Mumps may cause extraocular muscle palsies

Mumps is caused by a paramyxovirus that produces a fever and parotitis. Recent infection is characterised by a rise in antibody titre to the S antigen (antibody to the V antigen appears later but persists for many years). Sequelae of infection include orchitis, pancreatitis and meningoencephalitis. Ocular complications include dacryoadenitis and extraocular muscle palsies.

7.5 *Adenoviruses*

a. The adenoviruses are DNA viruses
b. Transmission is solely by airborne routes
c. There are approximately 20 serological types
d. Types 8 and 19 cause epidemic keratoconjunctivitis
e. Types 3 and 7 cause pharyngoconjunctival fever

The adenoviruses are a diverse group of DNA viruses—there are approximately 35 types. Transmission is mainly by the airborne route although faecal–oral transmission is common in children. The strains of interest to ophthalmologists are 8 and 19, which cause epidemic keratoconjunctivitis, and 3 and 7, which cause pharyngoconjunctival fever.

7.6 *Enteroviruses*

a. The enteroviruses are double stranded RNA viruses
b. They include the polioviruses
c. The main mode of spread in ocular infection is the faecal–oral route
d. Acute haemorrhagic conjunctivitis is caused by Entero 70 virus
e. Acute haemorrhage conjunctivitis is caused by Coxsackie B24

The enteroviruses are a family of single stranded RNA viruses that possess an icosahedral capsid. They are acid and bile stable and include the polioviruses (serotypes 1–3), Coxsackie (A1–A24, and B1–B6), and the echoviruses. The main route of transmission is faecal–oral, but direct contact and droplet spread are the more important modes in ocular infection. Acute haemorrhagic conjunctivitis (associated with overcrowding and poor hygiene in tropical and subtropical regions) is associated with the Coxsackie A24 and Entero 70 viruses.

8: Hepatitis B and HIV

8.1 Properties of the hepatitis B virus

a. It is a DNA virus
b. The Australia antigen is associated with the inner core
c. The HB "e" antigen is associated with the outer coat
d. Hepatitis B is transmitted vertically and horizontally
e. 5% of acute cases become long term carriers

Hepatitis B is a DNA virus that possesses an inner core and an outer protein coat. An excess of this protein coat produced by the liver cells is called the hepatitis B surface antigen or Australia antigen. The HB "e" antigen is associated with the inner core. Transmission of hepatitis B is predominantly horizontal (by parental inoculation or by sexual routes) but vertical transmission will occur from mothers to babies if the mother is "e" antigen positive. The virus has an incubation period of between 6 weeks and 6 months, and approximately 5% of acute cases become long term carriers.

8.2 *Serology of hepatitis B*

a. The HB surface antigen level is raised in the acute illness and in carriers
b. The HB surface antibody indicates past or present disease
c. Presence of the HB "e" antigen indicates acute infection or supercarriers
d. The HB core antibody is present in the blood of vaccinated people
e. Carriers of the HB "e" antibody should be classified as "high risk"

A knowledge of the serology of Hepatitis B is important when assessing the hepatitis state (past or present) of a patient. The level of HB surface antigen is raised in the acute illness, and if it remains raised for 6 months or longer the patient is by definition a carrier. Presence of the HB surface antibody may indicate that the patient has had the disease and is now immune or that they have been given the hepatitis B vaccine. The HB "e" antigen indicates acute infection or supercarrier status: such patients should be classified as high risk. Carriers of this antibody, although they should not be blood donors, pose no risk from needlestick injuries. The presence of the HB core antibody indicates that the patient has had the disease naturally and is not present in vaccinated people.

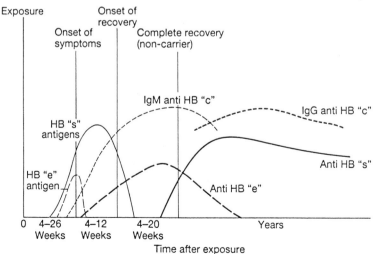

Fig 43 Serological changes in acute hepatitis B

8.3 *HIV*

> a. HIV is an oncogenic retrovirus
> b. HIV is a single stranded RNA virus
> c. HIV viruses are homogeneous
> d. HIV infection is completely exogenous
> e. HIV is killed by a pH below 1.0 or above 13

The human immunodeficiency virus (HIV) is a non-oncogenic cytocidal retrovirus. It contains a single strand of RNA and possesses the reverse transcriptase enzyme. AIDS viruses are not a homogeneous group: HIV-1 and HIV-2 differ in the make up of their glycoprotein envelopes. HIV infection is completely exogenous (unlike transforming retroviruses); these viruses do not contain any conserved cellular genes—nor do they cause infection by activating silent sequences in cellular DNA. HIV is not a particularly robust virus and is killed by strong acid and alkali (pH $\leqslant 1.0$ and $\geqslant 13$), and by exposure to 10% bleach or 50% ethanol.

8.4 *Pathogenesis of HIV infection*

> a. HIV is trophic for CD8 receptors
> b. HIV will cause T helper cells to form multinucleate giant cells
> c. HIV has a profound cytopathic effect on monocytes and macrophages
> d. HIV has no effect on humoral immunity
> e. HIV may become latent in monocytes

HIV is trophic for T helper lymphocytes, whose CD4 receptors act as receptors for the virus. Viral infection of T helper cells will produce a profound cytopathic effect, forming multinucleate cells and eventually causing cell death. Monocytes and macrophages also possess CD4 like receptors but viral infection rarely results in a profound cytopathic effect or cell death. By destroying T helper cells the virus cripples the cell mediated immune response, predisposing to viral, protozoan, and some neoplastic conditions. HIV can also effect the humoral immune response and is known to cause polyclonal antibody production, hypergammaglobulinaemia, and the production of autoantibodies (it will also cause a decrease in the production of T cell dependent immunoglobulins). HIV may become latent in monocytes and macrophages and be transported to sites such as the lungs and central nervous system. The body's immune response against HIV is hampered because the latent virus is "invisible" to immune defences, and its frequent mutations produce different glycoprotein envelopes—resulting in constantly changing antigenic stimuli.

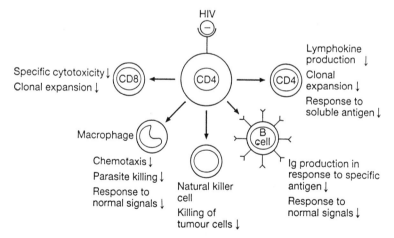

Fig 44 **Human immune system modulation by HIV infection of CD4 lymphocytes**

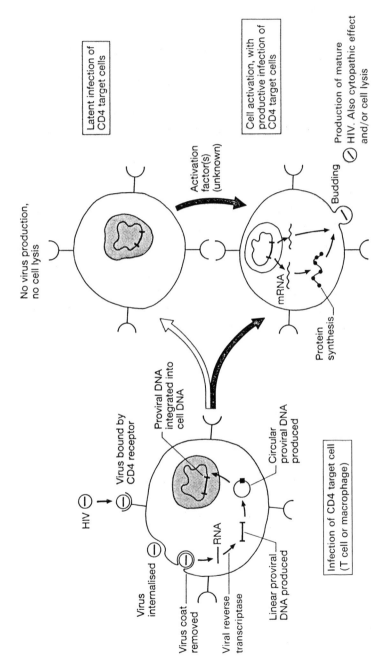

Fig 45 The life cycle of HIV

8.5 Serology of HIV

> a. Antibodies to envelope glycoproteins are present in ARC and AIDS
> b. Antibodies to the core protein are present in ARC and AIDS
> c. An increased T4/T8 ratio is seen in AIDS
> d. HIV may be grown in culture and isolated from lymphocytes from the peripheral blood
> e. ELISA is the most common diagnostic set for HIV

The profile of antibody response to HIV infection will vary between the AIDS related complex (ARC) and "fully blown" AIDS. Antibodies against envelope glycoproteins such as gp41, gp120, and gp160 are present in both the AIDS related complex and AIDS. Transition from the complex to AIDS is signalled by a decrease in antibody to core proteins such as p24, and a decrease in the T4/T8 ratio. HIV may be grown in culture with CD4 target cells and may be isolated from lymphocytes from the peripheral blood. ELISA is the most common diagnostic test currently in use.

8.6 Ocular manifestations of HIV

> a. CMV retinitis is seen in ARC
> b. Incidence of herpes simplex keratitis increases
> c. Cottonwool spots are the most common findings
> d. Incidence of toxoplasma chorioretinitis rises
> e. Incidence of candida chorioretinitis increases

CMV retinitis is seen only in fully blown AIDS and not in the AIDS related complex (ARC). It reflects the degree of immune suppression and is a grim prognostic indicator (mean survival after diagnosis is approximately 9 months, even with treatment). Cottonwool spots are the most common finding in AIDS; they are secondary to ischaemia, which causes interruption of axoplasmic flow. The incidence of herpes simplex keratitis is not increased (despite the increased incidence of chronic mucocutaneous infection with herpes simplex) nor of candida infection. Other opportunistic pathogens that are found include toxoplasma, histoplasmosis and herpes zoster. The incidence of toxoplasma chorioretinitis does not increase, but the incidence of brain abscesses related to toxoplasmosis does.

9: Fungi

9.1 *General properties of fungi*

> a. Fungi are heterotrophic
> b. Fungi function only as saprophytes
> c. Yeasts are unicellular fungi
> d. Moulds are characterised by mycelium
> e. Mycelia bear reproductive spores

Fungi are heterotrophic eukaryotic microorganisms; that is, they are dependent upon exogenous sources of organic food and must therefore function as saprophytes or parasites. Broadly speaking, fungi can be divided into two groups—the yeasts (which are unicellular), and the moulds (characterised by branching filaments known as mycelium). These mycelia absorb nutrients from the substrate and bear reproductive spores (which are characteristic for each species).

9.2 *Candida albicans*

> a. This is a normal commensal organism of the gastrointestinal tract
> b. Infection is usually exogenous
> c. Candida commonly causes oral and vaginal infection
> d. Presence of antibodies to candida is indicative of a deep seated infection
> e. Infection by *Candida albicans* can cause a retinitis

Candida albicans is the most common cause of human candidiasis. It is a normal commensal of the mouth and gastrointestinal tract and most infections are endogenous in origin. The most common infections are oral or vaginal but deep seated infection is seen in the immunosuppressed patient. The diagnosis of disseminated infection requires isolation from deep sites, blood, cerebrospinal fluid, or urine: the mere presence of antibodies is not indicative of a deep seated infection. *Candida albicans* can also cause a retinitis whose appearance is often mistaken for that of the cottonwool spots induced by ischaemia.

9.3 *Cryptococcus neoformans*

> This organism:
> a. Is a true pathogen
> b. Is a mould
> c. Is found in pigeon droppings
> d. Primarily causes lung infections
> e. May cause a chronic meningoencephalitis

Cryptococcus neoformans is a yeast whose normal habitat is the droppings of pigeons. It is a true pathogen and primarily causes lung infections (the droppings become dried and the yeast is inhaled). The organism may spread in the bloodstream to the meninges, where it gives rise to a chronic meningoencephalitis, which is fatal if untreated.

9.4 *Aspergillus fumigatus*

a. This is a true pathogen
b. Spores germinate in the bronchi, producing mycelium
c. Mycelial antigens cause Type I and Type II hypersensitivity reactions
d. Aspergillomas have an increased incidence in sarcoidosis
e. Neutropenia predisposes to deep infections

Aspergilli are common saprophytic fungi often found in decomposing plant debris, and their spores cause a number of different forms of aspergillosis if inhaled. *Aspergillus fumigatus* (the strain most commonly found in humans) is an opportunistic pathogen. The inhaled spores germinate in the lumen of the bronchi to form abundant mycelia, which may spark an IgE mediated allergic response (Type I hypersensitivity), and/or the production of IgG antibodies leading to complement activation and infiltration by polymorphs (Type II hypersensitivity reaction). An aspergilloma consists of a compact mass of mycelia and is found in lung cavities remaining after healed tuberculosis bronchiectasis or sarcoidosis. Invasive aspergillosis is a devastating infection often seen in immunocompromised patients, especially those who are neutropenic.

10: Protozoa

10.1 *Helminths*

a. Nematodes are flatworms
b. Filarias are all transmitted by biting insects
c. Trematodes all have fresh water snails as intermediate hosts
d. Cestodes are tapeworms living in the lumen of the gastrointestinal tract
e. *Toxoplasma gondii* is a helminth

The helminths may be divided into two broad groups: platyhelminths (or flatworms); nematodes (roundworms). The nematodes can be further divided into filariasis (which are all transmitted by biting insects), such as *Onchocerca volvulus*; and intestinal roundworms (such as *Ascaris lumbricoides*). The platyhelminths may be further divided into cestodes or tapeworms (including *Echinococcus granulosus*, which causes hydatid disease) and the trematodes or flukes (which all have fresh water snails as their intermediate hosts). The trematodes include *Schistosomiasis*. *Toxoplasma gondii*, although a protozoan, is not a helminth.

10.2 *Onchocerciasis*

a. Humans are the only definitive hosts
b. The disease is spread by mosquitoes
c. Infective larvae mature over 1 year in the skin
d. Systemic spread via the blood is the main route of ocular infection
e. The Mazzotti skin test detects infection

Onchocerciasis (commonly known as river blindness) is caused by *Onchocerca volvulus* and affects 30 million people worldwide. This condition is spread by the blackfly, and the only definitive hosts are humans. The blackfly picks up microfilariae from the skin which metamorphose to infective larvae in its thoracic walls. Infective larvae (which are transferred to humans who are bitten by the blackfly) mature in the skin for approximately 1 year, there being between 50 and 200 million microfilariae in the skin of a heavily infected individual. Systemic spread by the blood is unusual and the main route of ocular infection is from the nearby skin directly to the conjunctiva and cornea. The Mazzotti skin test (which involves injection of diethylcarbamazine) is used to detect infection.

10.3 *Toxocariasis*

a. *Toxocara catis* and *Toxocara canis* are parasites of the gastrointestinal tract
b. Infection is by ingestion of adult nematodes
c. Splenic involvement is common
d. Retinal lesions consist of a focal vasculitis with granulomas
e. The complement fixation test is the main diagnostic tool

Toxocariasis is caused by *Toxocara catis* and *Toxocara canis*, which are gastrointestinal parasites. Infection is by hand to mouth contact with eggs and larvae which, once in the digestive tract, pass transmurally to the lymph nodes and venules and hence to the spleen, lungs, eyes, and other sites. Ocular toxocariasis is characterised by retinal haemorrhage with focal vasculitis and granuloma formation but no necrosis. ELISA is the most sensitive and specific diagnostic aid for this condition.

10.4 *Cestode infections*

a. Cysticerosis is caused by *Taenia saginata*
b. Cysticerosis causes chronic retinal inflammation and fibrosis
c. *Echinococcus granulosus* causes hydatid disease
d. *Echinococcus granulosus* has humans as primary host
e. Schistosomiasis is a form of cestode infection

Cysticerosis is caused by the cestode *Taenia solium*, which is found in pork. The ingested larvae mature in the gut before multiplying and crossing the mucosa to enter the bloodstream and hence the retina. Retinal involvement is characterised by chronic inflammation and fibrosis and is often complicated by retinal detachments. *Echinococcus granulosus* is the causative organism of hydatid disease; its prevalence is higher in sheep farming communities. Humans (the primary host) are infected by swallowing ova from dog faeces. The larvae then pass to extraintestinal sites such as the liver to form hydatid cysts. Ocular involvement is often characterised by proptosis. Schistosomiasis is a trematode infection which rarely involves the eye, although a case of central retinal artery occlusion by *Schistosomiasis mansoni* has been reported.

10.5 *Properties of Toxoplasma gondii*

> a. This is an obligate intracellular parasite
> b. The human is the definitive host
> c. Transmission may occur via uncooked meats
> d. Congenital toxoplasma accounts for 50% of ocular disease
> e. Only antibody negative mothers are at risk of vertical transmission

Toxoplasma gondii is an obligate intracellular protozoan parasite whose definitive host is the cat. Transmission may occur by a number of routes including ingestion of uncooked meats (as almost all livestock, for example sheep, pigs and to a lesser extent cows can be infected), or by inhalation. Vertical transmission is also possible if an antibody negative mother is infected during pregnancy. The chance of congenital toxoplasmosis is increased if the maternal infection is in the third trimester, but the severity of the illness is greatest if the infection occurs in the first trimester. Congenital toxoplasmosis accounts for almost all toxoplasma eye disease.

10.6 *Life cycle of Toxoplasma gondii*

> a. Asexual merozoites are converted to gametocytes in the cat gut epithelium
> b. Fully infective sporozoites are excreted in cat faeces
> c. Bradyzoites rapidly divide in the intermediate host's gastrointestinal epithelium
> d. Extraintestinal cyst sites include skeletal muscle, heart, brain, and the eye
> e. Extraintestinal spread is often via white blood cells

As the cat is the definitive host of *Toxoplasma gondii* the conversion of the asexually produced merozoites to gametocytes can occur only in its intestinal epithelium. These microgametes will produce oocysts that are excreted in the faeces and spore in the soil after 1–5 days. The eggs will become fully infective only after sporulation and ingestion by an intermediate host, such as humans. The ingested sporozoites assume a rapidly dividing form (tachyzoite) before travelling to the lymph nodes, often protected inside white blood cells. Extraintestinal spread to skeletal muscle, the heart, brain, and the eye is common and cysts at these sites enclose the slowly dividing bradyzoites.

10.7 *Pathogenicity of Toxoplasma gondii*

a. The conoid is a primitive mouthpiece
b. Parasitophorous vacuoles are formed on entering the cell
c. Vacuoles are susceptible to lysozymal destruction
d. Cysts are destroyed by "naive" macrophages
e. The retina is a more common site of infection than the choroid

The first stage of infection is cell penetration, which is accomplished by the primitive mouthpiece or conoid (which contains a number of lytic enzymes). Once in the cell a parasitophorous vacuole resistant to lysozymal destruction is formed. The retina is infected in preference to the choroid because it possesses lower immunoglobulin levels. Cell mediated immunity utilising activated macrophages is the prime defence against toxoplasma infection.

10.8 *Acanthamoeba*

a. This is an aerobic microorganism
b. It will grow on a blood agar plate
c. Acanthamoeba stains with acridine orange
d. Infections may respond to neomycin
e. Infection is associated with use of extended wear contact lenses

Acanthamoeba is an aerobic organism that is difficult to culture, growing only on a non-nutrient agar with a killed *Escherichia coli* overlap. Identification may be aided by a number of stains including acridine orange and calcofluor white. Acanthamoebal infections are most commonly associated with soft and extended wear contact lenses, the mostly commonly isolated organisms being *Acanthamoeba polyphaga* and *Acanthamoeba castellani*. The resultant keratitis may require prolonged treatment with antibiotics such as neomycin, but oral regimens of ketoconazole and fluconazole have also proved effective.

11: Antimicrobial agents

11.1 *Properties of penicillins*

a. Penicillins inhibit cross linking of glycan strands in bacterial cell wall
b. They are bacteriostatic
c. These drugs are effective against Gram positive bacilli
d. Ampicillin is effective against most Gram negative bacilli
e. Flucloxacillin is susceptible to β lactamase

The penicillins are a large group of effective, bactericidal and generally non-toxic antibiotics that are produced from fungi and by molecular modifications. Penicillins achieve their action by interfering with the cross linking of glycan strands which is the final stage in the production of the bacterial cell wall. They are most effective against streptococci and Gram positive bacilli such as the clostridia. *Staphylococcus aureus* infections are commonly resistant, because their β lactamases destroy penicillin. The antibacterial spectrum of ampicillin has been extended to include Gram negative bacilli such as *Escherichia coli* and *Haemophilus influenzae*. The side chain of flucloxacillin prevents the action of staphylococcal β lactamase.

125

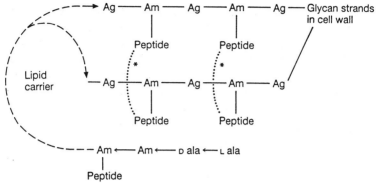

Fig 46 Mode of action of penicillins and cephalosporins. Am, Acetylmuramic acid; Ag, acetylglucosamine; ala, alanine; *site of penicillin and cephalosporin action on peptide cross linkages

11.2 Properties of cephalosporins

a. Cephalosporins inhibit folic acid production
b. They are bactericidal
c. Cefuroxime is a third generation cephalosporin
d. These drugs are effective against Gram negative bacilli
e. They are effective against β lactamase producing staphylococci

The cephalosporin family of antibiotics falls into the β lactamase category, exerting bactericidal effects by inhibiting cell wall synthesis. Most cephalosporins have a wider range of activity than penicillins, encompassing β lactamase producing staphylococci and Gram negative bacilli. Cefuroxime is a second generation cephalosporin effective against many Gram negative bacilli that are resistant to broad spectrum penicillins such as ampicillin. The Gram negative spectrum has been extended in third generation cephalosporins such as ceftazidime to include *Pseudomonas* and *Bacteroides*.

11.3 Properties of gentamicin

a. This drug prevents the first ribosome joining with messenger RNA
b. It is bacteriostatic
c. Gentamicin is effective against streptococci and anaerobes
d. It has little effect on Gram negative bacilli
e. Ototoxicity is more common than renal toxicity

Gentamicin is from the aminoglycoside group of bactericidal antibiotics. It exerts its actions at the site of the ribosome by preventing the first ribosome from joining with messenger RNA; it may also cause the messenger RNA code to be misread so that the wrong amino acid is incorporated into the protein. Most aminoglycosides are effective against staphylococci and aerobic Gram negative bacilli, including *Pseudomonas* and resistant *Proteus* strains. They are felt to be ineffective against streptococci and anaerobic bacteria. If administered parenterally gentamicin is known to cause vestibular, cochlear, and renal side effects (in decreasing order of frequency).

11.4 *Properties of the tetracyclines*

Tetracycline:
a. Disrupts cell wall synthesis
b. Is bacteriostatic
c. Is effective against chlamydia
d. Is effective against *Brucella abortus*
e. Is contraindicated in pregnancy

Tetracyclines interrupt the cycle of attachment of amino acids to the first binding site during protein synthesis. They are bacteriostatic agents with a wide spectrum that includes Gram positive cocci, aerobic Gram negative bacilli and bacteroides. They are also the treatment of choice in chlamydial infections such as trachoma and the more unusual infections such as brucellosis and Q fever. Tetracyclines have a number of common side effects such as disturbance of the gut, and are contraindicated in pregnancy.

11.5 *Properties of chloramphenicol*

Chloramphenicol:
a. Inhibits protein synthesis
b. Is bactericidal
c. Has a broad spectrum, including staphylococci
d. May cause aplastic anaemia
e. Causes the "grey baby" syndrome

Chloramphenicol is a potent, potentially toxic, broad spectrum antibiotic. Its bacteriostatic action is achieved by preventing the transfer of the growing peptide chain to other amino acids, thus inhibiting protein synthesis. It is commonly used topically for bacterial conjunctivitis because of its potency against staphylococci. Its systemic use, however, should be limited to the treatment of life threatening conditions such as *Haemophilus influenzae* meningitis or thyroid fever because of its potentially fatal side effect of aplastic anaemia. It may also cause the "grey baby" syndrome in neonates and is therefore contraindicated in pregnancy and when breast feeding.

11.6 *Properties of metronidazole*

a. This drug affects DNA synthesis
b. It is effective against anaerobes
c. It is effective against giardia
d. Resistance is a problem
e. Use of metronidazole may disrupt liver function tests

Metronidazole exerts its antimicrobial effect by disrupting DNA synthesis. It is effective against many anaerobic bacteria such as bacteroides and is often used as a prophylaxis for gastrointestinal surgery. It is also effective against protozoan parasites such as giardia, trichomonas and entamoeba. Resistance is not a problem as yet and side effects are uncommon, although disrupted liver function tests and low platelet counts have been reported.

11.7 *Properties of amphotericin*

a. This drug binds to sterols in cell membranes
b. It may be administered orally
c. Amphotericin has a narrow fungal spectrum
d. Renal toxicity is common
e. Anaemia is a known side effect

Amphotericin is still the standard antimicrobial agent and until recently was the only drug used for the treatment of deep mycoses. This polyene is not absorbed from the gut—therefore it must be administered intravenously. The drug binds to sterols in cell membranes, and its selective activity is due to its very high affinity for ergosterol (the major sterol in fungal membranes). Its antimicrobial spectrum includes most fungi that invade humans. Common side effects include anaemia and renal toxicity.

11.8 *Other antifungal agents*

a. Flucytosine is effective in cryptococcosis
b. Flucytosine penetrates poorly into the CSF
c. Flucytosine has a low incidence of resistance
d. Ketoconazole may cause fatal liver damage
e. Ketoconazole is useful in chronic mucotaneous candidiasis

Flucytosine has a limited spectrum, including candidiasis or cryptococcosis. Its major advantage is that it well absorbed orally and penetrates into the cerebrospinal fluid very easily. However, there is a high incidence of resistance to this drug which may be avoided if it is given in combination with amphotericin B. Ketoconazole is also active after oral administration but it has been known to cause fatal liver damage and its use should be limited to conditions such as chronic mucotaneous candidiasis.

11.9 *Resistance to antibiotics*

a. Gene mutation induces resistance to antituberculous drugs
b. Transduction involves passage of genetic material in plasmids
c. Conjugation employs bacteriophages
d. Aminoglycosides are destroyed by acetylation
e. Resistance may be achieved by modifying the target of antibody attack

Resistance to antimicrobial agents may arise in a number of ways. Gene mutation is a mechanism that is important only in the antituberculous drugs such as rifampicin and antifungals such as flucytosine. More important mechanisms involve gene transfer from one bacterium to another—by transduction (genetic material is incorporated into a bacteriophage and later into the genome of another cell), or by conjugation (the direct passage of genetic material using a plasmid from one cell to another). Exposure to some of the new cephalosporins has been shown to activate previously dormant or weak resistance mechanisms in certain organisms. The genetic changes may convey resistance by:

1. destroying or inactivating the drug (e.g. acetylation of aminoglycosides)
2. excluding the antibiotic
3. modifying the target site (e.g. failure of ribosomes to bind erythromycin)
4. using alternative enzymic pathways that are resistant to the drug (e.g. enzymes resistant to sulphonamide and trimethoprim).

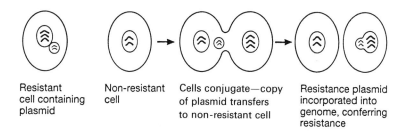

Resistant cell containing plasmid

Non-resistant cell

Cells conjugate—copy of plasmid transfers to non-resistant cell

Resistance plasmid incorporated into genome, conferring resistance

Fig 47 **Mechanisms of resistance to antimicrobial agents**

11.10 *Properties of acyclovir*

a. This drug is a guanosine analogue
b. Unaltered, it inhibits viral DNA polymerase
c. Acyclovir is effective against herpes simplex and varicella zoster viruses
d. Its use may cause renal insufficiency
e. Resistance arises by viral mutation

Acyclovir, which is an acyclic analogue of guanosine, is an extremely safe and effective antiviral agent, and is the drug of choice for most forms of herpes simplex and varicella zoster virus (VZV) infections. Acyclovir itself is inactive and inhibits viral DNA polymerase only after phosphorylation by viral thymidine kinase. Because it is so selective—it has affinity only for viral thymidine kinase—it is effective only in infected cells. It may be administered orally, parenterally or topically. Common side effects include a mild renal insufficiency, gastrointestinal upset and headache. The most common cause of resistance to acyclovir is a mutation resulting in the loss of viral thymidine kinase synthesis, but acyclovir resistant HSV and VZV mutants are uncommon in immunocompetent patients.

11.11 *Properties of ganciclovir*

a. Ganciclovir is a nucleotide analogue
b. Is active against cytomegalovirus
c. Is as effective against herpes simplex as acyclovir
d. Should be administered orally
e. Neutropenia and thrombocytopenia are rare side effects

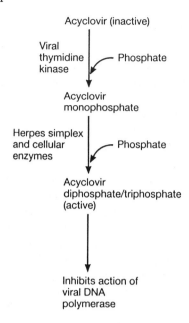

Fig 48 **Mechanism of action of acyclovir**

Ganciclovir is an acyclic nucleotide analogue, differing from acyclovir in that it has a terminal hydroxymethyl group. Its triphosphate form appears to function both as an inhibitor of and as a faulty substrate for cytomegalovirus DNA polymerase (host cell polymerase is much less sensitive to it). It is 10–25 times more active than acyclovir against cytomegalovirus and at least as active against herpes simplex and VZV. Ganciclovir is poorly absorbed from the gut and so must be given intravenously. Treatment of CMV retinitis involves an induction course followed by maintenance therapy, because ganciclovir has only a virostatic action. The reported adverse effects of the drug have been mainly haematological, primarily neutropenia (in 40% of patients) and thrombocytopenia (20% of patients).

11.12 *Properties of foscarnet*

a. Foscarnet is a nucliodide analogue
b. It reversibly inhibits the viral DNA polymerase and reverse transcriptase
c. It has an intrinsic anti HIV effect
d. It is active against cytomegalovirus
e. This drug causes renal insufficiency and neutropenia

Foscarnet is paraphosphate analogue of phosphonoacetic acid that selectively and reversibly inhibits viral specific DNA polymerases and reverse transcriptases. Foscarnet appears to be about as effective as ganciclovir for the initial 2–3 week induction therapy of CMV retinitis and, because of its mode of action, is effective in treating acyclovir resistant herpes simplex infections. It is of particular use in the AIDS patient because it is thought to have an intrinsic anti HIV activity and may be used in conjunction with zidovudine without the risk of catastrophic neutropenia. Common side effects include renal insufficiency and proteinuria.

Answers

1.1	a, b, e	3.2	a, c, e	5.2	a, c, e		
1.2	a, b, d	3.3	a, b, e	5.3	b, c, e		
1.3	b, c, d	3.4	a, c, d, e	5.4	a, b, c, d, e		
1.4	a, b, d, e	3.5	b, c, e	5.5	a, b, d, e		
1.5	a, b, d	3.6	a, c, e	5.6	a, b, d, e		
1.6	a, b, c, d, e	3.7	a, c, d	5.7	a, c, d		
1.7	a, b, e	3.8	a, c, e				
1.8	a, b, c, d	3.9	a, b, c, d, e			6.1	c, d, e
1.9	a, b, e	3.10	b, d, e			6.2	a, c, d
		3.11	a, b, c, e			6.3	a, c
2.1	a, b, e					6.4	a, d, e
2.2	a, c, d, e	4.1	a, b, d			6.5	a, b, d
2.3	c, d, e	4.2	a, c, e			6.6	b, c, d, e
2.4	c, d, e	4.3	a, c, d			6.7	a, b, c, e
3.1	a, b, d	5.1	a, b			7.1	a, c, e

7.2	a, b, e	**9.2**	a, c, e	**11.2**	b, d, e
7.3	a, b, c, e	**9.3**	a, c, d, e	**11.3**	a, e
7.4	a, c, d, e	**9.4**	b, c, d, e	**11.4**	b, c, d, e
7.5	a, d, e			**11.5**	a, c, d, e
7.6	b, d	**10.1**	b, c, d	**11.6**	a, b, c, e
		10.2	a, c, e	**11.7**	a, d, e
8.1	a, d, e	**10.3**	a, c, d	**11.8**	a, d, e
8.2	a, c	**10.4**	b, c, d	**11.9**	a, d, e
8.3	b, d, e	**10.5**	a, c, e	**11.10**	a, c, d, e
8.4	b, e	**10.6**	a, d, e	**11.11**	a, b, c
8.5	a, d, e	**10.7**	a, b, e	**11.12**	b, c, d
8.6	c	**10.8**	c, d, e		
9.1	a, c, d, e	**11.1**	a, c, d		

Pathology

1: Inflammation

1.1 *General characteristics of acute inflammation*

Acute inflammation:
a. Is a specific response
b. Exhibits memory
c. Comprises a cellular followed by a vascular phase
d. May be caused by chemical injury
e. May be present for 1–2 weeks

Acute inflammation may be defined as the non-adaptive response of viable vascular tissue to subfatal injury. Unlike the immune response, which is adaptive, acute inflammation is non-specific and does not exhibit memory (the acute inflammatory response will not be quicker and more pronounced on the second exposure to a stimulus). The causes of acute inflammation include infection, trauma, ultraviolet light, X ray radiation and chemical injury. By definition, acute inflammation lasts only 1–2 days and comprises a vascular phase followed by a cellular phase.

1.2 *Vascular phase of acute inflammation*

a. Vasodilatation is initiated by histamine
b. Kinins will vasodilate capillaries and venules
c. Prostaglandin E$_2$ constricts arterioles
d. There is a decreased vascular permeability
e. Axial streaming is present

The vascular phase is initiated by a number of chemical mediators. Histamine, which is released from degranulated mast cells, produces an increase in vascular permeability and will vasodilate venules—peak effect is reached after 5 minutes. The effect of histamine is only transient (approximately 15 minutes) but kinins will also cause capillaries and venules to dilate and their release along with prostaglandins such as prostaglandin E_2 (PGE_2) (which dilates arterioles) produces a delayed and persistent vascular response. Such a response has a peak effect at approximately 4–24 hours. As a result of vasodilatation, blood flow becomes slower and cells move to the sides of the vessels—an effect known as axial streaming.

1.3 Cellular phase of acute inflammation

> a. Neutrophils predominate
> b. The negative charge of neutrophils is increased
> c. Migration occurs through endothelial cells
> d. Macrophages constitute a second cellular wave
> e. Is stimulated by chemotactic factors

Neutrophils make up 40–75% of the circulating white cells and have a characteristic segmented nucleus with a granular cytoplasm. The initial wave of the cellular response is predominantly neutrophils. Owing to axial flow the neutrophils (which are heavier than red cells) come to lie at the periphery of the blood column and some adhere to the endothelium—this is known as margination. Adhesion of neutrophils to the endothelium is increased because the negative charge of neutrophils (that normally repels them from negatively charged endothelial cells) decreases on exposure to certain chemotactic factors. Adherent neutrophils put out pseudopodia, which enter the gaps between adjacent endothelial cells so facilitating their passage into the perivascular space. The biphasic pattern of cell accumulation is completed by a second wave of macrophages. All of these changes occur under the influence of chemotactic factors.

136

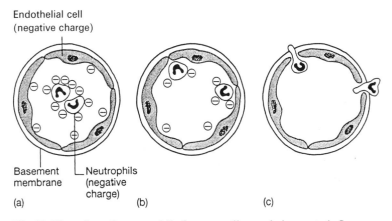

Fig 49 Migration of neutrophils from small vessels in acute inflammations: (a) Normal small vessel; (b) margination of neutrophils and decreased negative charge; (c) pseudopodia inserted between endothelial cells and neutrophils penetrate the basement membrane

1.4 *Chemotaxis*

> a. Chemotaxis is the directional and purposive movement of phagocytic cells
> b. It occurs along a concentration gradient
> c. Polymorphs have specific chemotactic binding sites
> d. C3b is a chemotactic factor
> e. Increase of intracellular cyclic AMP stimulates chemotaxis

Chemotaxis is the directional and purposive movement of phagocytic cells towards areas of tissue injury or bacterial invasion. Chemotaxis may be divided into two phases: reception of chemotactic signals; and the cellular response to these signals, known as transduction. Many substances are known to be chemotactic for neutrophils, and may be classified into three groups: (1) low molecular weight compounds such as prostaglandin E; (2) intermediate molecular weight compounds (such as C5a and C5 derived peptides); (3) high molecular weight compounds (e.g. lymphokines and partly denatured proteins).

Chemotaxis follows a concentration gradient of such factors, which have specific binding sites on the polymorph. Binding of these factors will cause an influx of calcium by stimulating phospholipase A_2. This in turn stimulates arachidonic acid metabolism with the subsequent activation of guanosyl cyclase and an increase in levels of cyclic GMP, which will increase microtubule assembly and so aid polymorph migration. A rise in cyclic AMP will inhibit tubule assembly and chemotaxis.

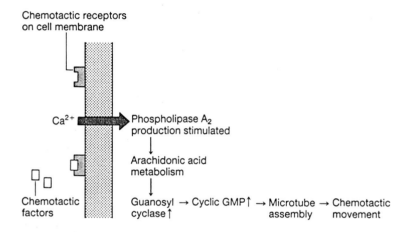

Fig 50 The transduction phase of chemotaxis

1.5 *Phagocytosis*

a. C3b aids recognition
b. Bacteria are engulfed in a phagosome
c. A "respiratory burst" is essential for killing cells
d. Myeloperoxidase increases the bactericidal capacity of hydrogen peroxide
e. Lactoferrin is employed in killing cells

The initial stage of phagocytosis (recognition) is aided by the process of opsonisation. Two of the most important opsonins are IgG and complement C3b. Polymorphs have specific receptor sites for these molecules, which attach themselves to invading microorganisms. The bacterium or foreign object is then engulfed by a phagosome. The phagosome fuses with a lysosome; this is associated with a burst of metabolic activity (the respiratory burst), which results in the production of hydrogen peroxide. The killing action of hydrogen peroxide is increased 50-fold by the action of myeloperoxidase which is found in lysosomes. Other methods of cell killing include lowering the pH, lysosomal hydrolysis and production of lactoferrin (which inhibits the growth of some microorganisms).

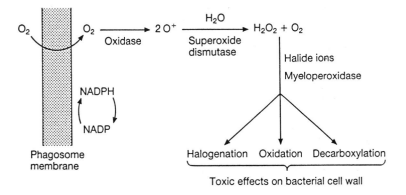

Fig 51 Oxygen dependent bacterial killing

1.6 *Properties of macrophages*

Macrophages:
a. Are derived from monocytes
b. Are incapable of division
c. Are activated by complement C3b
d. Fuse to form epithelioid cells
e. Are important in antigen presentation

139

Macrophages are derived from monocytes within the tissues by a process that involves enlargement of the cell, and increase in lysosome numbers, and development of a more prominent golgi apparatus and endoplasmic reticulum. One of the factors involved in macrophage activation is C3b. Macrophages are capable of cell division and in the face of persistent foreign material may fuse to form multinucleated giant cells with increased phagocytotic activity. Epithelioid cells (usually found in granulomas) evolve from a single macrophage and have increased secretory capacities.

1.7 *Properties of activated macrophages*

Activated macrophages may:
a. Have greater capacity to kill tumour cells
b. Produce endogenous pyrogen and interferon
c. Inhibit proliferation of fibroblasts and polymorphs
d. Secrete lymphokines
e. Have increased phagocytic capacity

Activation of macrophages has a number of consequences: the phagocytotic capacity of the macrophage is increased, hydrolytic enzymes are produced; activated macrophages are capable of producing endogenous pyrogen and interferon (which blocks translation of viral messenger RNA). Macrophage activation also has a number of effects on other inflammatory and immune cells—for example, it stimulates the proliferation of fibroblasts and its colony stimulating factor increases polymorph production. Macrophages secrete a lymphocyte activating factor (interleukin-1), which will stimulate T helper cells. Lymphokines (such as macrophage chemotactic factor and migration–inhibition factor) are secreted by T helper cells to aid recruitment of macrophages to the sites of infection.

1.8 *The complement system*

a. C3a and C5a are anaphylatoxins
b. C3a has greater activity than C5a
c. C567 is chemotactic to polymorphs
d. Plasmin stimulates the classical and alternative pathways
e. C5b6789 causes cell lysis

The complement system is involved in acute inflammation, phagocytosis, clotting, immune, and hypersensitivity reactions. It may be initiated by the classical or alternative pathways, both of which are stimulated by plasmin. C3a and C5a will increase vascular permeability and are chemotactic for polymorphs—they are known as the anaphylatoxins. C5a is approximately 1000 times more active than C3a. C567 is also chemotactic to polymorphs but only the killing complex of C5b6789 is capable of cell lysis.

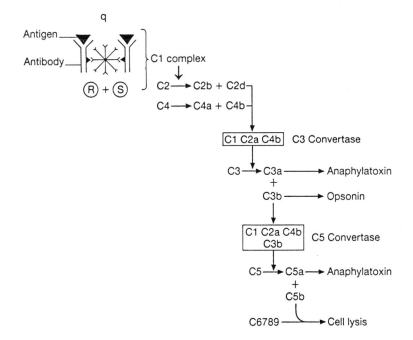

Fig 52 The classical complement pathway

1.9 *Kinin, clotting and fibrinolytic systems*

> a. Active Hageman factor stimulates the kinin cascade
> b. Active Hageman factor inhibits plasminogen
> c. The kinin cascade produces potent vasoconstrictors
> d. Fibrinopeptides stimulate vascular leakage
> e. Plasmin activates Hageman factor

Inflammatory mediators derived from the plasma include the kinin system, the clotting system and the fibrinolytic system. Activated Hageman factor will stimulate all three cascades by its stimulatory action on factor XI, prekallikrein, and plasminogen. The kinin cascade will produce a number of potent vasodilators, including bradykinin. Fibrinopeptides produced by the clotting cascade are chemotactic for neutrophils and will stimulate vascular leakage. Positive amplification loops exist within all three systems: activated factor XI, kallikrein, and plasmin all feed back positively to activate Hageman factor.

1.10 *Natural history of inflammation*

> a. Resolution may occur after tissue destruction
> b. Organisation produces normal structure
> c. Regeneration produces normal structure
> d. Regeneration is dependent on cell type
> e. Lost tissue is replaced by vascularised connective tissue

The natural history of an acute inflammatory lesion depends upon a number of factors. If the inflammatory response does not result in tissue destruction, and exudate is fully removed by polymorphs, the result is resolution. If the exudate persists it will become organised to produce scarring. If the inflammatory condition causes tissue destruction, regeneration (return to the original state) can occur only if the cells lost had been labile cells (which divide and proliferate throughout postnatal life), or stable cells (which, although normally quiescent, may be stimulated to divide). If tissue derived from permanent cells (which proliferate only during fetal life) is destroyed it cannot be replaced, and a scar comprising vascularised connective tissue is formed.

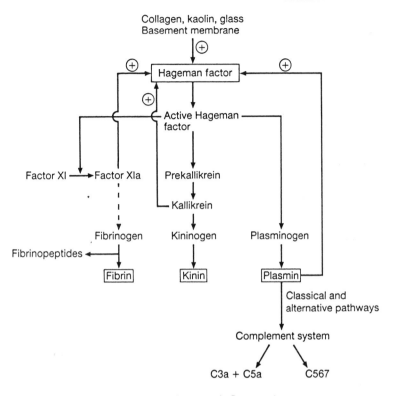

Fig 53 Plasma cascade systems in acute inflammation

1.11 *Wound healing*

a. Proliferation of epithelial cells is stimulated by chalones
b. Fibronectin stimulates epithelial migration
c. New vessels appear within 24 hours
d. Fibroblasts produce collagen and glycosaminoglycans
e. Myofibroblasts cause wound contraction

Wound healing involves both epidermal and dermal events. In the epidermis epithelialisation occurs in three stages: (1) cell migration, which is stimulated by fibronectin; (2) cell proliferation, normally inhibited by chalones; and (3) differentiation. Dermal events involve the invasion of the fibrin clot by solid buds of endothelial cells, which grow from intact capillaries at the wound edges and form new vessels within the first week.

143

Macrophages and fibroblasts then migrate into the wound; macrophages aid clot removal while fibroblasts produce collagen and glycosaminoglycans. Myofibroblasts will appear at the wound edges in the first week and are thought to be responsible for wound contraction.

1.12 *Properties of chronic inflammation*

Chronic inflammation:
a. Has vascular and cellular phases
b. Is always infectious in origin
c. Is characterised by granuloma formation
d. Polymorphs predominate
e. Always arises from areas of prolonged acute inflammation

Chronic inflammation is caused by the presence of a persistent and particulate irritant. It is characterised by a cellular response, during which cellular proliferation and destruction (mostly of macrophages and macrophage derived cells) occur simultaneously. These cells are often organised in a special type of chronic inflammation known as a granuloma. Although infections such as tuberculosis and leprosy are common causes of chronic inflammation, the origin is not always infective (for example, sutures, silica, and wood granulomas). Non-specific chronic inflammatory conditions may arise from acute inflammatory lesions, but the specific granulomatous response seen in tuberculosis has a very transient acute phase.

1.13 *Properties of tuberculous granuloma*

Tuberculous granuloma:
a. Has an inner core of lymphocytes and microorganisms
b. Contains epithelioid cells with an increased phagocytic capacity
c. Contains multinucleate giant cells
d. Is a caseating granuloma
e. Has an outer layer of fibroblasts

A granuloma may be defined as a lesion arising from a special type of chronic inflammation, mostly of macrophage and macrophage derived cells. The tuberculous granuloma consists of an inner core of microorganisms and epithelioid cells with increased secretory capacity (secondary to prominent Golgi apparatus and rough endoplasmic reticulum). This core is surrounded by a layer of activated macrophages (which have ingested the bacilli) and a layer of T lymphocytes. The outer layer consists of fibroblasts and multinucleate giant cells, although in "young granulomas" the giant cells may be found in the central core. Caseation is a typical feature of tuberculous granulomas.

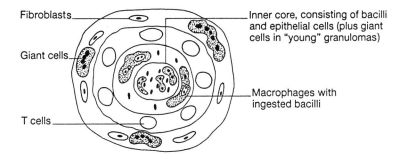

Fibroblasts — Inner core, consisting of bacilli and epithelial cells (plus giant cells in "young" granulomas)

Giant cells —

T cells — Macrophages with ingested bacilli

Fig 54 Tuberculous granuloma ("old")

2: Immunology

2.1 B and T lymphocytes

> a. Plasma cells are derived from B lymphocytes
> b. T lymphocytes cannot produce antibodies
> c. B cells produce chemotactic factors for macrophages
> d. B cells are found in the paracortical zones of lymph nodes
> e. T cells have surface receptors for Fc and C3b

Both B and T lymphocytes are derived from bone marrow stem cells. B lymphocytes will mature into plasma cells that are capable of antibody production, and are the mainstay of the humoral immune response. T cells are incapable of antibody production but are able to synthesise and secrete a number of active components known as lymphokines. These activate macrophages, which (along with T cells) form the basis of the cell mediated immune response. These two classes of lymphocytes have a different distribution within the secondary lymphoid tissue, B cells being found in the cortical follicles of lymph nodes and T cells in the paracortical zones. There are no morphological differences between the two but the cells possess a number of different surface markers—the Fc and C3b receptors are found only on B cells.

2.2 Immunoglobulins

> a. Immunoglobulins have two heavy and four light chains
> b. Heavy chains determine the type of immunoglobulin
> c. The Fc fragment binds antigen
> d. The chains are held together with disulphide bonds
> e. Each chain has a "variable" and a "constant" domain

Antibodies (or immunoglobulins) when in the monomeric form all have the same basic Y shaped structure consisting of four polypeptide chains held together by disulphide bonds. Each monomer has a pair of identical heavy chains and a pair of identical light chains, each of which has a "variable" and "constant" domain. The immunoglobulin type is determined by the constant region of the heavy chains, there being five classes: γ, α, μ, δ, and ε. There are two classes of light chain: κ and λ. Each immunoglobulin monomer has two fragment antigen binding (Fab) sites, located at the variable regions of the light and heavy chains. The third fragment of the monomer has no power to bind antigen and is known as the fragment crystallisable (Fc) site; however, it is capable of complement activation and immune adherence to neutrophils and macrophages.

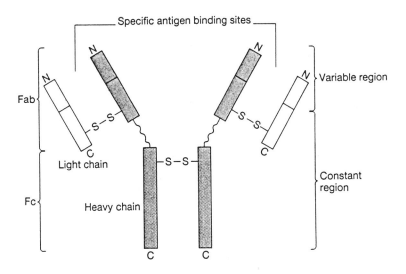

Fig 55 Basic immunoglobulin structure

2.3 *Immunoglobulin types*

a. IgG accounts for 70–80% of plasma immunoglobulins
b. IgM crosses the placental barrier easily
c. IgM is a strong complement activator
d. IgA is a dimer found in seromucus secretions
e. IgE binds via its Fab portion to mast cells

There are five classes of immunoglobulin: IgA; IgD; IgE; IgG; IgM. IgG counts for 70–80% of plasma immunoglobulins, is a monomeric structure, and functions as an important opsonin and complement activator. IgM is the largest immunoglobulin and is a pentameric structure with ten potential antigen binding sites (however, only five of these are usually involved at any one time). Because of its size IgM does not cross the placental barrier but its pentameric structure renders it a strong complement activator. IgA appears selectively in seromucus secretions of the gastrointestinal and respiratory tracts as well as in tears, sweat, bile, and breast milk. It has a dimeric structure with linkage being achieved by a J chain. The Fc portion of IgE binds to receptors on mast cells and cross linkage of Fab portions by antigen will result in mast cell degranulation. IgD (found on the surface of 50% of B lymphocytes) is the least common immunoglobulin.

2.4 Function of the immunoglobulins

Immunoglobulins are involved in:
a. Neutralisation of bacterial toxins
b. Prevention of bacterial and viral cell entry
c. Opsonisation
d. Complement activation via the alternative pathway
e. Stimulation of natural killer cells

Immunoglobulins may function in a number of ways:
(1) Neutralisation of bacterial toxins. This is important in infections such as tetanus, diphtheria and cholera
(2) Opsonisation. Here the Fab fragment binds to the bacterial cell wall and phagocytosis is mediated via the Fc receptors on the surface of neutrophils
(3) Complement activation. Immunoglobulins (especially IgG and IgM) activate complement by the classical pathway and so cause cell lysis
(4) Antibody dependent cell mediated cytotoxicity—the activation of lymphocytes known as natural killer cells by immunoglobulins
(5) Prevention of foreign antigen penetration across mucosal surfaces. IgA molecules bind to bacteria and viruses, preventing them from adhering to mucosal surfaces of the gastrointestinal and respiratory tracts) entering the tissues.

2.5 *Properties of the major histocompatibility complex*

a. MHC class I antigens are found in all cells
b. MHC class II antigens are found predominantly in macrophages
c. T helper cells have CD4 receptors for MHC class II antigens
d. Cytotoxic T cells have CD8 receptors for MHC class I antigens
e. T cells bind to the polymorphic part of MHC antigens

The major histocompatibility complex (MHC) is a set of genes, located on the short arm of chromosome 6, which code for cell surface glycoproteins, which are of great importance in "self" recognition. The two types of MHC antigens differ in structure, function and distribution. MHC type I antigens are coded for by HLA A, B, and C gene sequences and are found in all cells except red blood cells. These cells will process "endogenous" antigens (e.g. viral peptides produced by an infected cell) and present them in conjunction with MHC class I antigens on their surface membranes. Type II MHC antigens are classified by HLA D sequences, and are found predominantly on macrophages, Langhans' cells, dendritic cells, and occasionally on cells that have been exposed to γ interferon. These phagocytic cells ingest "exogenous" antigens (e.g. bacterial antigens), which are then "processed" and presented together with MHC class II antigens on their surface membranes. T cells are capable of recognising foreign antigen only in association with MHC antigens; they therefore possess receptors for the monomorphic section of MHC antigens. T cells can, broadly speaking, be divided into two groups: (1) CD4 cells, which recognise foreign antigen in association with MHC class II antigens (MHC class II restricted); (2) CD8 cells, which recognise foreign antigen in association with MHC class I antigens (MHC class I restricted). Originally it was thought that CD4 cells corresponded to T helper cells and CD8 cells to suppressor and cytotoxic T cells but there now appears to be a degree of CD4 "heterogeneity," with some cells possessing "suppressor" activity.

2.6 *Function of T cells*

> a. T cells are the predominant cell type in cell mediated immunity
> b. T helper cells release lymphokines
> c. T helper cells aid antibody production
> d. Cytotoxic T cells can kill viruses
> e. T cells produce γ interferon

T cells are the predominant cell type in cell mediated immunity. Once T helper cells have been stimulated by antigen presenting macrophages they release lymphokines, including interleukins 4–6 which stimulate B cells (to which the same antigens have bound) to proliferate and mature. T cells may also produce interleukin 2, a lymphokine that stimulates cytotoxic T cell activity and antibody production. Cytotoxic T cells are able to kill viruses and virus infected cells directly or by the production of γ interferon. These cells play an important role in immunity against protozoal and helminth infection.

2.7 *Cytokines*

> a. Interleukin 1 produced by macrophages stimulates T helper cells
> b. Cytotoxic T cells are activated by interleukin 2
> c. Interleukins 4 and 5 stimulate B cells
> d. B cells produce macrophage activating factor
> e. The production of some cytokines is increased by γ interferon

Cytokines are inducible hormone like polypeptides which act via specific protein receptors and often have multiple biological effects. Included in this group are lymphokines (produced by T cells), monokines (produced by polymorphs and macrophages), interleukins (which may be produced by either of the above), and γ interferon. Interleukin 1 is produced by macrophages; it stimulates the clonal expansion of T helper cells and increases their production of interleukin 2. Interleukin 1 has numerous other actions including its role as endogenous pyrogen. T helper cells will produce interleukin 2, which is predominantly involved in the activation of cytotoxic T cells and the non-MHC restricted natural killer cells. Interleukin 2 also aids antibody production by B cells (in conjunction with interleukins 4 and 5). T cells also produce a number of lymphokines (such as macrophage activating factor and migration inhibition factor) that modulate macrophage activity. γ Interferon is not produced only in antiviral states; it also plays an important role in immune regulation with actions synergistic with interleukin 2 (such as regulation of macrophage and cytotoxic T cell function). The production of γ interferon is influenced by interleukins 1, 2, 4, 6, and tumour necrosis factor α(TNFα).

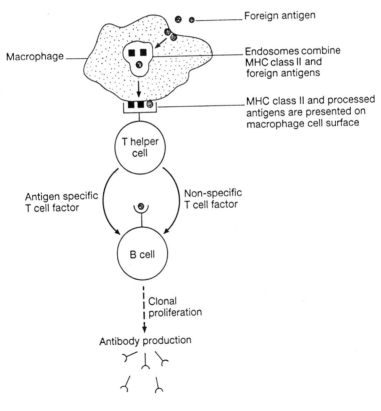

Fig 56 Production of T cell dependent antibody

151

2.8 *Immunity to viruses*

a. Direct killing by cytotoxic T cells is the most important factor
b. Phagocytosis by polymorphs is common
c. Interferons inhibit viral replication
d. All antiviral antibody activity is dependent on T cells
e. Interferons stimulate natural killer activity

The prime defence of the body against viral infection is direct killing of the virus by cytotoxic T cells that recognise foreign viral antigen in association with MHC type 1 antigens. Another important method is phagocytosis by activated macrophages. All antiviral antibody activity is T cell dependent: it aids viral destruction in conjunction with complement. Interferons (cell regulatory glycoproteins) are produced in response to viral infections, especially double stranded RNA viruses. They induce an antiviral state by synthesising proteins that inhibit viral replication and may increase non-specific killing by natural killer cells. Interferons are also thought to play an important role in the immune response to neoplasia.

2.9 *Important factors in immunity to protozoa*

a. Killing of protozoa by cytotoxic T cells
b. Stimulation of eosinophils by T cells
c. Eosinophil mediated antibody dependent cell mediated cytotoxicity
d. Production of histaminase by eosinophils
e. T cell mediated increase in gastrointestinal mucus secretions

Cytotoxic T cells play a relatively small role in immunity against protozoan infection—eosinophils are especially prominent in the immune response against worms. Worm antigen will

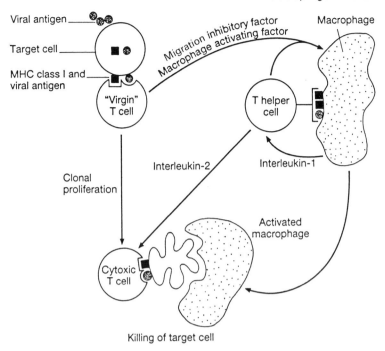

Fig 57 **Viral immunity**

stimulate T cells to produce eosinophil stimulation promoter and this, along with eosinophil chemotactic factors produced by the worms (and by degranulating mast cells), draws activated eosinophils to the site of infection. There the eosinophils have a twofold effect, which includes antibody dependent cell mediated cytotoxicity and control of the inflammatory process by production of histaminase. Expulsion of nematodes from the gut is accomplished by an increase in mucus gastrointestinal secretions (caused by non-specific T cell factors) that stick to and debilitate the worms, which are then expelled.

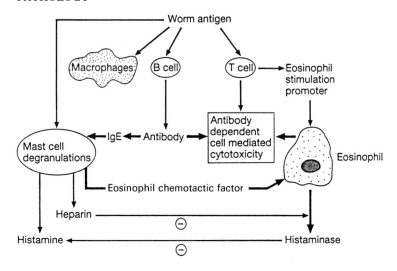

Fig 58 Eosinophils in protozoan immunity

3: Hypersensitivity reactions

3.1 *Type I hypersensitivity*

a. This follows contact with an allergen
b. Cross linkage of IgE Fab fragments causes mast cell degranulation
c. C3a and C5a cause degranulation
d. Mast cells contain histamine, 5 HT and heparin
e. Histamine stimulates mast cell degranulation

A hypersensitivity reaction may be defined as an adaptive immune response that has occurred in an exaggerated or inappropriate form. Type I hypersensitivity is an "allergic" reaction that immediately follows contact with an antigen which would normally not cause a marked immune response (an allergen). The basic mechanism of type I hypersensitivity is mast cell degranulation, caused by cross linkage of IgE molecules on mast cell surfaces via their Fab fragments, by C3a and C5a complement fragments, or by certain drugs such as codeine and morphine. Mast cell degranulation results in release of histamine, 5 HT, heparin, eosinophil chemotactic factors, and platelet activating factors. Histamine exerts negative feedback on this reaction to inhibit mast cell degranulation.

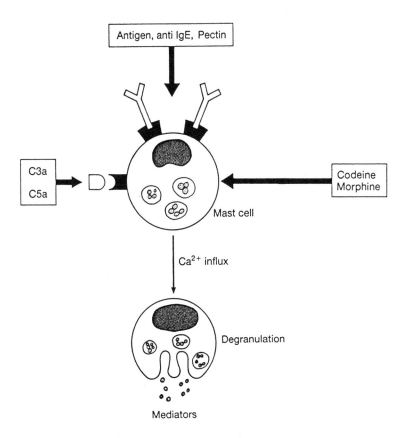

Fig 59 Mast cell activation

3.2 *Type II hypersensitivity*

a. This is caused by circulating immune complexes
b. Tissue damage is induced by phagocytes
c. It is characterised by the Arthus reaction
d. Rhesus incompatibility is an example of type II hypersensitivity
e. Hyperacute graft rejection is an example of type II hypersensitivity

Type II hypersensitivity is caused by antibody directed against cell surface or tissue antigens which interact with complement and other inflammatory systems. Tissue damage is caused by "frustrated" phagocytes, which are unable to ingest the whole tissue and so release their lysosomal contents. Examples of type II hypersensitivity include rhesus incompatibility of the newborn, in which IgG against rhesus D antigen is produced by rhesus negative mothers and crosses the placenta to attack the red cells of the rhesus positive fetus. ABO incompatibility (mismatched transfusion) is also an example, as is "hyperacute" graft rejection. The Arthus reaction is characteristic of type III hypersensitivity reactions.

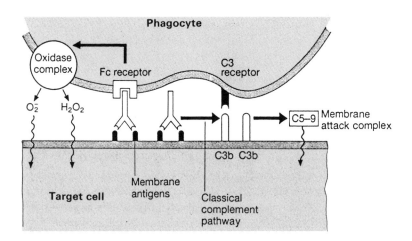

Fig 60 Type II cytotoxic mechanisms

3.3 Type III hypersensitivity

a. This is caused by antibody directed against cell surface antigens
b. It stimulates an acute inflammatory reaction in the tissues
c. Turbulence of blood flow may determine site of disease
d. Type III hypersensitivity is uncommon in autoimmune diseases
e. It may be caused by chronic infection

Type III hypersensitivity reactions are caused by the deposition of immune complexes in tissues which then stimulate complement activation, so producing an acute inflammatory reaction. Common causes of type III hypersensitivity reactions include persistent infections (e.g. viral hepatitis), and autoimmune disease (e.g. rheumatoid arthritis). Type III hypersensitivity is dependent on the persistence of these immune complexes, but the more important factor is their deposition which is governed by:

● haemodynamics—increased turbulence of blood flow (as seen in the glomerulus, choroid plexus and ciliary body) stimulates deposition;
● increased vascular permeability secondary to histamine;
● specific antigen tissue binding, where the antigen–antibody complex is specific to a single organ.

The Arthus reaction is seen after antigen is intradermally injected into individuals whose circulating antibody levels are high because of previous immunisation. The antigen–antibody complex is then deposited, resulting in an acute inflammatory reaction that peaks at 4–10 hours.

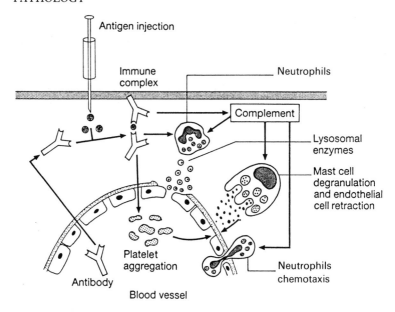

Fig 61 Type III hypersensitivity: the Arthus reaction

3.4 *Type IV hypersensitivity*

a. This may develop within 12 hours of exposure to allergen
b. It is transferable in serum
c. It includes contact dermatitis
d. Type IV hypersensitivity may be produced by subdermal injection of tuberculin
e. The granulomatous type peaks at 48 hours

Type IV hypersensitivity (also known as cell mediated hypersensitivity) is of four types, all involving T cells and therefore not transferable in serum. They include all those hypersensitivity reactions that take more than 12 hours to develop.

(a) The Jones–Mote type is produced by stimulation of basophils and peaks at 24 hours
(b) Contact dermatitis is characterised by an epidermal reaction consisting of mononuclear cells (but no polymorphs) and peaks at 48 hours

158

(c) Tuberculin type hypersensitivity is caused by subdermal injection of tuberculin producing a reaction in the dermis that peaks at 48–72 hours (the Heaf test)

(d) Cell mediated hypersensitivity results in a granulomatous reaction, and is usually caused by persistent antigen in macrophages (e.g. tuberculosis). This reaction peaks at approximately 4 weeks.

4: Transplantation immunology

4.1 *Tolerance*

a. Clonal "abortion" of B cells causes tolerance
b. B cell "exhaustion" produced by persistent antigenic stimulation is a cause of tolerance
c. Functional deletion of T helper cells causes tolerance
d. Development of T cell tolerance is less rapid than B cell tolerance
e. T cell tolerance is more persistent than B cell tolerance

Medewar's experiments on mice were instrumental in defining the concept of tolerance, which may be defined as the development of non-reactivity towards a particular antigen. There is now thought to be a spectrum of tolerance, ranging from antigen induced responsiveness (partial or low zone tolerance) to antigen induced unresponsiveness (complete or high zone tolerance). Experimental studies have shown that T cell tolerance is induced more rapidly than B cell tolerance (1 day versus 7 days) and by lower antigen concentration. T cell tolerance persists for up to 6 months, whereas B cell tolerance lasts less than 2 months. Exposure of immature B cells to monomeric antigen inhibits the development of cells with that antigenic specificity—this is known as clonal "abortion". A similar mechanism is thought to occur with immature T cells, and both result in high zone tolerance. Low zone tolerance (involving the deletion of only some aspects of the immune system) may be achieved by a number of means: high concentrations of antigen may reduce the responsiveness of T and B cells (clonal "anergy"); T cells may undergo functional deletion or be suppressed by T suppressor cells; T helper cell deletion/suppression may produce a degree of B cell tolerance by disrupting the production of T cell dependent antibodies.

4.2 *Types of transplantation*

> a. Autografts are taken from the patient
> b. Grafts between all twins are isografts
> c. Allografts are not genetically identical
> d. The species of donor and recipient differ in xenografts
> e. The most common allografts are kidneys

Transplantation may be defined simply as the transfer of a graft from a donor to a recipient. There are several types of transplantation, including autografts (which are taken from the patient him- or herself), isografts (which occur between identical twins), allografts (the donor and recipient are of the same species but are not genetically identical), and xenografts (where the donor and recipient are not of the same species). The most common allografts are blood transfusions.

4.3 *Tissue typing*

> a. Typing is carried out for all HLA subtypes
> b. Matching for MHC class II antigen is more important than for MHC type I antigen
> c. "Sensitivity" is greater in women than in men
> d. "Sensitivity" is decreased by recurrent blood transfusions
> e. HLA mismatch accounts for late onset rejection

The major histocompatibility complex antigens HLA class I (A, B and C) and class II (D subtypes) are those recognised by the body's immune surveillance system and are therefore important in transplant rejection. Tissue typing is carried out only for HLA subtypes A, B, and DR loci. It is of primary importance to accurately match the DR locus, as even a single mismatch significantly increases the incidence of graft rejection. Well matched transplants have a 15% greater survival at 1 year than transplants that are not well matched. However, after this initial phase transplants are lost from both groups at the same rate and so HLA mismatching may not account for late onset rejection. The phenomenon of "sensitivity" is seen more commonly in women than men (because of pregnancy) and in those who have received multiple blood transfusions or previous transplants. Highly sensitised patients will benefit from meticulous HLA matching.

4.4 *Types of rejection*

a. Hyperacute rejection occurs in minutes
b. Accelerated rejection is predominantly cell mediated
c. Acute rejection occurs within 7 days
d. Acute rejection is antibody mediated
e. Acute on chronic rejection is found only in immunosuppressed patients

Rejection may be defined as a series of changes that result in the destruction of the graft as a functioning entity. The terminology used to describe types of graft rejection is often confusing, but a simple knowledge of the body's response to foreign antigens will clarify matters. If circulating antibodies are present to antigens found on the graft hyperacute rejection (characterised by complement activation, polymorph infiltration, and thrombus formation) will occur within minutes. If the recipient has been sensitised to donor antigen memory cells will be stimulated (T and B cells), which leads to graft destruction (predominantly by cell mediated mechanisms). This accelerated rejection occurs within 2–5 days. Acute graft rejection is predominantly cell mediated and occurs at 7–21 days—it is an allogenic reaction to donor antigen. Rejection occurring after 3 months is termed as chronic and occurs as a result of disturbing post graft tolerance. Antibodies and complement are the main mediators in pure chronic rejection: T cells are the main instigators of acute on chronic rejection (which is found only if the recipient's immune system has been altered—in immunosuppression).

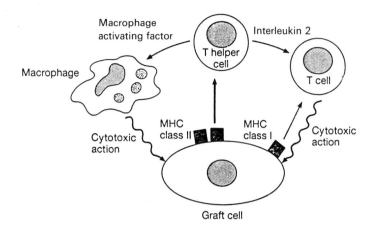

Fig 62 Graft cell destruction

5: Cardiovascular pathology: thrombosis

5.1 *Platelet structure*

a. The peripheral zone is rich in glycoproteins
b. The sol-gel zone contains platelet factor 3
c. α Granules contain factor VIII related antigen
d. α Granules contain ADP
e. The dense tubular system is found in the membrane zone

Platelets may be divided into four zones: peripheral, sol-gel, organelle, and membrane zones. The peripheral zone is rich in glycoproteins essential for the platelet adhesion and aggregation reactions. This layer also contains platelet factor 3, which accelerates the clotting process during platelet aggregation. The sol-gel zone contains microtubules and microfilaments, which help maintain the discoid shape of the platelet. The organelle zone contains α granules (whose constituents include factor VIII related antigen, factor V, fibrinogen, fibronectin, platelet-derived growth factor, and chemotactic factors), and other granules known as dense bodies (containing ADP, calcium and 5HT). The inner, membrane, zone is connected to the surface by an open canalicular system and contains the dense tubular system responsible for platelet contractile functions and prostaglandin synthesis.

5.2 *Thrombus formation*

a. Platelet adhesion is stimulated by exposure to basement membrane collagen
b. Calcium released from dense tubules stimulates granule release
c. The granule release reaction is stimulated by prostaglandins E_1 and I_2
d. Platelet aggregation is stimulated by ADP and thrombin
e. Platelet aggregation is stimulated by prostaglandin I_2

The initial stage of thrombus formation, stimulated by exposure to endothelial collagen and to fibrin, is adhesion of platelets to vessel endothelium. Adhesion causes calcium release from the dense tubular system, which in turns leads to a change in the shape of the platelets and the release of granules. When the platelets are quiescent calcium is maintained at low levels by the operation of a cyclic AMP calcium pump. Antiaggregatory prostaglandins E_1, D_2, and I_2 act by stimulating adenylate cyclase (so increasing cyclic AMP). Aggregation follows platelet adhesion and is stimulated by ADP and thrombin. During aggregation platelets stick to one another to form a clump. Aggregation is stimulated by the vasoconstrictive agent thromboxane A_2 and is inhibited by prostaglandin I_2.

163

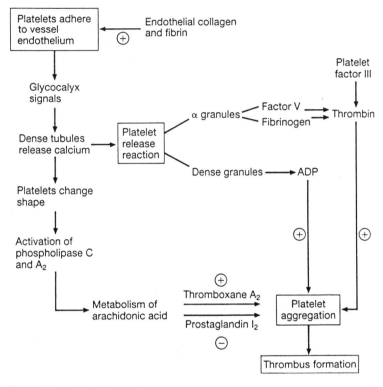

Fig 63 Thrombus formation

5.3 *Risk factors for thrombosis*

These include:
a. Venous stasis
b. Arrhythmias
c. Atherosclerosis
d. Type II hyperlipidaemia
e. Thrombocytopenia

Virchow described a triad of conditions that predispose to thrombus formation:
(1) a change in the nature of blood flow, such as venous stasis, cardiac arrhythmias, or valve disease;
(2) a change in the vessel wall caused by atherosclerosis, trauma, inflammation, or neoplastic change;

(3) a change in the constituents of the blood—an increase in the number of platelets or altered platelet function such as that seen in type II hyperlipidaemia (platelets are more sensitive to ADP and thrombin in this condition).

5.4 *Natural history of thrombi*

a. Thrombi may become detached from the vessel wall
b. They may be lysed by plasmin
c. Recanalisation occurs in mural thrombi
d. Thrombi may become covered with smooth muscle cells
e. Mural thrombi are infiltrated by blood vessels from the vasa vasorum

Thrombi have a varied natural history. They may become detached from the vessel wall, forming an embolus, or may be lysed by plasmin. If a thrombus persists it will become organised—this process will vary according to the site of thrombus formation. Occlusive thrombi in vessels may be replaced by a solid plug of collagenous tissue, or flow may be re-established by recanalisation. Mural thrombi are eventually covered by a proliferative layer of smooth muscle cells (which has been stimulated by the release of platelet derived growth factor) and this mass becomes vascularised by blood vessels derived from the main lumen of the vessel (not from the vasa vasorum).

5.5 *Forms of emboli*

Emboli come in several forms:
a. Thrombotic
b. Fluid
c. Nitrogen
d. Atherosclerotic
e. Fat

An embolus may be defined as an abnormal mass of material, transported in the bloodstream from one part of the circulation to another, which finally impacts in the lumen of a vessel through which it cannot pass. Emboli may be solid, fluid, and gaseous. The most common emboli are solid (for example, those caused by dislodged thrombus, atherosclerotic, tumour, and fat emboli). Amniotic fluid embolus is a rare obstetric complication. Gaseous emboli occur when air is introduced into the systemic circulation (such as by inadvertent opening of a large vein in head and neck surgery). Nitrogen emboli occur in decompression sickness (the "bends").

6: Cardiovascular pathology: atherosclerosis

6.1 Formation of atherosclerotic plaque

a. Endothelial cell trauma is a primary step in formation of plaque
b. Accumulation of intracellular lipid increases
c. Accumulation of extracellular lipid is increased
d. Platelets inhibit intimal proliferation
e. Plaques have the same topographical distribution as fatty streaks

The initial protagonists in the debate over the aetiology of atherosclerotic plaques were Virchow and Rokitansky, who proposed the "infiltrative" and "thrombotic" theories respectively. Endothelial damage is now believed to be the primary step in plaque formation. Platelets adhere to the injured endothelium and stimulate intimal smooth muscle proliferation by releasing platelet derived growth factor. Endothelial cell barrier function is now lost and accumulation of intracellular and extracellular lipid increases. Whether fibrolipid plaques are derived from fatty streaks (which may be seen from the age of 10–11 months) is uncertain—evidence against this association includes their different topographical distributions, and the triglyceride:cholesterol ratios of these two lesions.

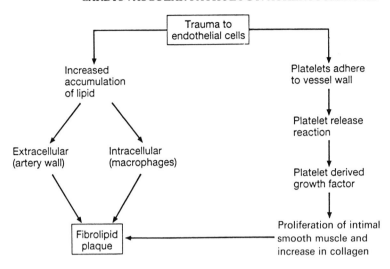

Fig 64 Atherosclerotic plaque formation

6.2 *Characteristics of fibrolipid plaques*

a. Thickening of the intima
b. Lipid laden macrophages
c. A smooth muscle layer underlying the lipid pool
d. Thickening of the adventitia media
e. Basal necrosis

The fibrolipid plaque is an elevated lesion that exhibits intimal thickening caused by proliferation of smooth muscle cells. This smooth muscle layer overlies a pool of lipid rich tissue debris (atheroma), which contains many lipid laden macrophages. Necrosis and softening at the plaque base is a common sequela, as is aneurysm formation caused by thinning of the adventitia media.

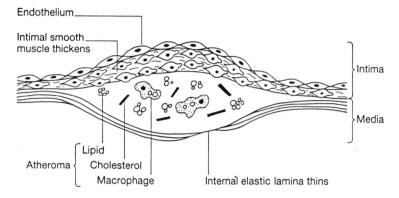

Fig 65 Atherosclerotic plaque

6.3 *Natural history and complications of atherosclerosis*

Sequelae of atherosclerotic plaques include:
a. Platelet microthrombi
b. Plaque fissures
c. Intraplaque haemorrhage
d. Aneurysm
e. Regression

The sequelae of atherosclerotic plaques may be uncomplicated or complicated. Included in the first group are simple plaque growth leading to a decrease in lumen size, and aneurysm formation caused by media thinning. Complicated plaques may arise by formation of plaque fissures caused by softening of the plaque base, or by intraplaque haemorrhage. In the first case small fissures will result in platelet microthrombi, and larger fissures in "dumb-bell" thrombi which may be occlusive or embolise. Atherosclerotic plaques are not thought to regress, but some studies have reported that vigorous dietary control has improved the angiographic pictures of peripheral vascular disease.

6.4 *Risk factors for atherosclerosis*

> These include:
> a. Smoking
> b. Age
> c. Diabetes
> d. Hypertension
> e. Raised levels of high density lipoprotein

Risk factors for atherosclerosis may be divided into two groups: reversible and non-reversible. Irreversible factors include age, male sex (but the increased incidence in men diminishes with age), and race. The most important reversible risk factors are cigarette smoking (risk of dying from a myocardial infarction is trebled if 15 cigarettes are smoked per day; this decreases in those who give up smoking), hypertension, diabetes mellitus, and hyperlipidaemia. Levels of high density lipoprotein are inversely related to the risk of coronary heart disease because it takes up free cholesterol from extrahepatic tissues.

7: **Neoplasia**

7.1 *The cell cycle*

> a. Mitosis occupies most of the cell cycle
> b. Cell maturation occurs in G1
> c. The length of the cell cycle is determined by the S phase
> d. DNA synthesis occurs in the S phase
> e. The S phase is followed by mitosis

The cell cycle is made up of a number of phases, the first of which is mitosis (the M phase). This phase occupies only 1–2 hours; after this the daughter cells enter a gap phase (known as G1), during which cell maturation and differentiation occurs. G1 may last for days or years, depending on the tissue type, and is the main determinant of the length of the cell cycle. After G1 the cells enter the S phase in which DNA synthesis occurs. This phase lasts approximately 7–12 hours and is separated from mitosis by a second gap phase (G2), which lasts 1–6 hours.

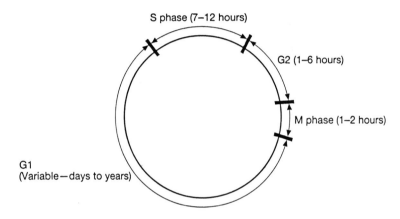

Fig 66 The cell cycle

7.2 *Characteristics of neoplasia*

a. Uncoordinated cell growth
b. Hyperplasia
c. A disturbance in cellular differentiation
d. Hypertrophy
e. Disturbance in the relationship between cells and surrounding stroma

The definition of a neoplasm (as suggested by Willis) is "an abnormal mass of tissue, the growth of which exceeds and is uncoordinated with that of the normal tissues, and which persists in the same excessive manner after cessation of the stimulus which has evoked the change." Characteristically neoplasms display a disturbance in cell proliferation, cell differentiation, and in the relationship between cells and their surrounding stroma. Both hyperplasia (an increase in the number of cells) and hypertrophy (an increase in the size of the cells) are adaptive conditions—that is, the excess growth will stop after the stimulus that evoked the change has ceased. They cannot therefore be classed as neoplastic conditions.

7.3 *Characteristics of dysplasia and metaplasia*

a. Metaplastic cells are poorly differentiated
b. Dysplastic cells are poorly differentiated
c. Chronic irritation is a stimulus for metaplasia
d. Invasion through the basement membrane is seen in dysplasia
e. Dysplasia is common in squamous epithelia

Metaplasia may be defined as a complete change in the differentiation of a cell from one fully differentiated form to another. It often arises as a response to chronic irritation and the transition is usually from a cuboidal or columnar epithelium to a squamous epithelium. Tumour metaplasia (such as adenocarcinomas of the lung changing to squamous carcinomas) has also been noted. Dysplastic conditions will display undifferentiated cells and abnormal mitoses but they are not invasive and do not pass through the basement membrane. Dysplasia often arises in a squamous epithelium—if the full thickness of the epithelial covering shows dysplastic change this is known as carcinoma in situ.

171

7.4 *Characteristics of malignant neoplasm*

These include:
a. Loss of differentiation
b. An increased number of abnormal mitoses
c. Nuclear pleomorphism
d. Non-invasiveness
e. A tendency to metastasise

Malignant neoplasms tend to be poorly differentiated, the cells being larger than their normal counterparts with a greater degree of heterogeneity in size and shape. The size of the nucleus is also variable and it tends to occupy a greater proportion of the total cell volume, increasing the nuclear:cytoplasmic ratio. The overall number of mitoses increases and the frequency of abnormal mitoses with tripolar, quadripolar or annular spindles higher. Malignant neoplasms will display invasiveness, in which cells separate and grow in an irregular pattern into the surrounding tissue. However, some "benign" lesions such as meningiomas and pleomorphic adenomas may be invasive. Cells entering the blood or lymphatic vessels and spreading to distant sites is known as metastasis.

7.5 *Mechanisms of neoplasia formation*

a. Loss of contact inhibition
b. Increased chalone production
c. Increased platelet derived growth factor production
d. Increased growth factor receptors
e. Increased beta transforming growth factor

Normal cell division ceases once contact is made with a neighbouring cell (contact inhibition). Contact inhibition is thought to occur by a negative feedback between cells, possibly via molecules known as chalones. One hypothesis for neoplastic growth is that chalone production is decreased, leading to excess cell division; another hypothesis is that surface membrane glycoproteins (which have been implicated in the control of contact inhibition) are changed in some way. Autocrine growth factors such as platelet derived growth factor and epidermal growth factor may cause neoplastic change if there is an increase in growth factor production, an increase in the number of growth factor receptors, or an exaggerated response to receptor stimulation. The beta transforming growth factor is an autocrine peptide that has a negative effect on cell growth and is thought to have a role in regulating cell population and size.

7.6 *Mechanisms of invasion*

a. Loss of adhesiveness
b. Increased fibronectin production
c. Loss of anchorage dependence
d. Collagenase trauma to basement membranes
e. Increased fibrin production

For metastasis to occur tumour cells must be shed from the original tumour mass (this may occur as a result of decreased adhesiveness between cells). Cell adhesiveness may decrease because of a deficiency of desmosomes, an increased net negative charge of some tumour cells, or the decreased production of fibronectin (which normally acts as an adhesive protein in cell to cell binding). Most cell growth requires a firm surface (anchorage dependent growth). This is not a feature of tumour cells, which may grow in suspension or in semisolid media. Invasion requires that neoplastic cells penetrate the interstitial stroma and basement membranes (this is aided by collagenases, which are present in a number of neoplastic cells such as breast carcinoma). Direct spread is also aided by plasminogen activator, which conveys an antifibrinolytic action to neoplastic cells.

7.7 Metastasis

a. Metastases are continuous with the primary growth
b. Metastasis occurs by lymphatic and blood borne spread only
c. Fibrin protects tumour emboli
d. Only 1% of emboli survive more than 24 hours
e. Site of metastasis is determined primarily by anatomical factors

A metastasis is a growing colony of malignant cells that becomes established at a point distant from the original or primary lesion, with which it has no continuity. The first step of formation is liberation of neoplastic cells, which then invade blood vessels or lymphatics (transcoelomic spread is also possible). These tumour emboli spread to distant sites but only 1% survive the initial 24 hours. Certain primary tumours preferentially metastasise to certain sites (Ewing and Paget suggested that different tumour cells would thrive in certain "biological soils" but not in others). Recent experiments using mouse melanoma cells have shown that cells destined to form secondary deposits in a particular organ can detach from their initial impaction site and "home in" on the favoured tissue. This homing property is thought to be related to the nature of the surface membrane of the malignant cells.

7.8 Oncogenesis: genetic factors

a. Down's syndrome predisposes to haematological malignancies
b. Xeroderma pigmentosum is a multiple gene abnormality
c. Familial polyposis is autosomal recessive
d. 40% of retinoblastomas are inherited
e. Klinefelter's syndrome predisposes to lung carcinoma

Genetic factors linked with oncogenesis may be due to chromosomal abnormalities—such as Down's syndrome (predisposing to acute myeloblastic and acute lymphoblastic leukaemias) and Klinefelter's syndrome (predisposing to breast carcinoma). Single gene abnormalities include xeroderma pigmentosum, which is an autosomal recessive condition that causes a defect in endonuclease excision and repair mechanisms of DNA, predisposing to squamous cell and basal cell carcinomas. Familial polyposis (another single gene abnormality) is transmitted in an autosomal dominant fashion. Because of an absence of an oncogenic suppressor gene on chromosome 13, 40% of all retinoblastomas are inherited.

7.9 Chemical carcinogens

The following are chemical carcinogens:
a. 3, 4 benzpyrene
b. 2-naphthylamine (which is an "ultimate" carcinogen)
c. Nitrosamines, which are "remote" carcinogens
d. Cyclophosphamide
e. Arsenic

A carcinogen may be defined as any factor that will increase an individual's chance of developing a malignant neoplasm. All chemical carcinogens are mutagens, that is they induce a permanent change in cell phenotype. Polycyclic hydrocarbons make up a large group of chemical carcinogens. Included in this group is 3, 4 benzpyrene, which is metabolised to a diol epoxide that covalently binds DNA and is highly mutagenic. Aromatic amines used in the textile and aniline dye industries (such as 2-naphthylamine) are "remote" carcinogens that become carcinogenic only after hydroxylation in the liver. Nitrosamines (also "remote" carcinogens) have been implicated in gastric carcinoma. Direct alkylating agents (such as cyclophosphamide), naturally occurring agents (such as aflatoxin), and occupational chemicals (such as arsenic) are all chemical carcinogens.

7.10 *Properties of oncogenes*

> a. Oncogenes disrupt cell cycle control
> b. Proto-oncogenes inhibit cell division
> c. Oncogenes are not naturally occurring
> d. They inhibit angiogenesis
> e. Oncogenes are found in some viral genomes

Oncogenes are naturally occurring genes that are involved in cell cycle control and interactions between the cell and its environment. A simple model for their role in carcinogenesis is that two levels of disregulation are involved in the cellular control of growth. The first of these is disruption of the cell cycle, which may be caused by activation of "dominant" proto-oncogenes that stimulate cell division, or by the loss of "recessive" suppressor genes that inhibit cell division. The second level is an alteration of the cell environment in ways that favour cell growth and dissemination. This may be achieved by the deletion of recessive suppressor genes responsible for the inhibition of angiogenesis. Oncogenic sequences have been found in the human papillomavirus (cervical carcinoma), Epstein–Barr virus (nasopharyngeal carcinoma and Burkitt's lymphoma) and hepatitis B virus (hepatoma).

7.11 *Activation of oncogenes*

> Oncogenes may be activated by:
> a. Point mutations in an oncogene
> b. "Promotor" gene insertion by viruses
> c. Oncogenic translocation
> d. Mutation of suppressor genes
> e. Deletion of suppressor genes

There are three basic mechanisms for oncogene activation.
(1) A point mutation in an oncogene may cause amplification of the oncogene "product" or an altered "product" with increased activity.

(2) Sections of the genome, known as promotor genes, may cause activation if they are inserted close to an oncogene (naturally occurring viruses). Oncogenes may also be inserted "downstream" from an active promoter: the Epstein–Barr virus causes a translocation of an oncogene to such an unsafe area, resulting in Burkitt's lymphoma.

(3) Inactivation of a recessive suppressor gene by mutation, deletion or translocation. Such genes include the retinoblastoma gene Rb1, and p53 (which has been implicated in lung, colonic and breast carcinoma).

Answers

1.1	d	**2.6**	a, b, c, d, e	**5.5**	a, b, c, d, e
1.2	a, b, e	**2.7**	a, b, c, e		
1.3	a, d, e	**2.8**	a, c, d, e	**6.1**	a, b, c
1.4	a, b, c	**2.9**	b, c, d, e	**6.2**	a, b, c, e
1.5	a, b, c, d, e			**6.3**	a, b, c, d
1.6	a, c, e	**3.1**	a, b, c, d	**6.4**	a, b, c, d
1.7	a, b, d, e	**3.2**	b, d, e		
1.8	a, c, d, e	**3.3**	b, c, e	**7.1**	b, d
1.9	a, d, e	**3.4**	c, d	**7.2**	a, c, e
1.10	c, d			**7.3**	b, c, e
1.11	b, d, e	**4.1**	a, b, c, e	**7.4**	a, b, c, e
1.12	c	**4.2**	a, c, d	**7.5**	a, c, d
1.13	c, d, e	**4.3**	b, c	**7.6**	a, c, d
		4.4	a, b, d, e	**7.7**	c, d
2.1	a, b			**7.8**	a, d
2.2	b, d, e	**5.1**	a, c, e	**7.9**	a, c, d, e
2.3	a, c, d	**5.2**	a, b, d	**7.10**	a, d, e
2.4	a, b, c, e	**5.3**	a, b, c, d	**7.11**	a, b, c, d, e
2.5	b, c, d	**5.4**	a, b, d		

Pharmacology

1: Pharmacokinetics

1.1 *Cornea*

> a. The epithelium is hydrophilic
> b. Epithelial phospholipids may retard drug penetration
> c. Active transport mechanisms account for transstromal drug movement
> d. The stroma is hydrophobic
> e. The endothelium is a greater barrier than the epithelium to drug transport

The corneal epithelium is a hydrophobic layer, containing anionic and cationic phospholipids, that may retard drug penetration. All drug transport through the cornea is by diffusion and no movement is possible against an electrochemical gradient. The stroma is hydrophilic and although the endothelium is hydrophobic the stroma and the aqueous may be considered as one pharmacokinetic "compartment" because the endothelium has such a low resistance to penetration by drugs.

1.2 *Intraocular drug transport*

> a. Breakdown of the blood aqueous barrier increases drug inactivation
> b. Pigment binding of drugs increases their efficacy
> c. Pigment binding increases the duration of action of atropine
> d. Excretion of drugs is mainly via transscleral spread
> e. Drugs may be actively transported from the vitreous

The iris, ciliary body, lens, and vitreous can be considered as one pharmacokinetic "compartment". Breakdown of the blood aqueous barrier will increase the protein concentration in the aqueous, resulting in accelerated drug inactivation. Binding of drugs such as atropine and pilocarpine to pigment decreases their efficacy but increases their duration of action. Excretion of drugs from the aqueous is mainly via the trabecular meshwork but penicillin like drugs may be actively transported from the vitreous to the retina.

1.3 *Bioavailability of corticosteroids*

a. Corneal penetrance is increased if drug preparations are biphasic
b. Phosphate preparations penetrate the inflamed eye well
c. Fluoromethalone has very marked corneal penetrance
d. Topical administration is more efficacious than periocular injection for anterior chamber penetrance
e. Intravitreal injection increases the efficacy of steroid therapy

The ideal topical preparation should be biphasic so that it can pass through the hydrophilic and hydrophobic layers of the cornea: acetate solutions are like this. Phosphate preparations penetrate the inflamed eye well but have markedly lower anti-inflammatory actions than acetate preparations. Fluorometha-lone has very limited corneal penetrance and therefore is useful for long term treatment, because its use decreases the risk of raising intraocular pressure. Penetrance of corticosteroids applied topically into the anterior chamber is better than that achieved by periocular injections, which are usually reserved for cases of severe uveitis. As corticosteroids are removed rapidly from the vitreous, intravitreal injections are seldom worthwhile.

2: Cholinergic agonists

2.1 The ocular cholinergic system

a. Cholineacetyl transferase is found in the corneal epithelium and the retina
b. Acetylcholine is found in the corneal stroma and endothelium
c. Cholinesterase is found in the iris and ciliary body
d. Cholinesterase is found in the retinal vessels
e. Muscarinic receptors are found in the epithelium

Cholineacetyl transferase (the enzyme responsible for acetylcholine production) is found in the corneal epithelium, the iris ciliary body, and inner plexiform layer of the retina. Acetylcholine and cholinesterase are also found in these sites: the latter in particularly high concentrations in the iris and ciliary body sphincter muscles. However, cholinesterase is not found in the primary aqueous, the vitreous, or the retinal vessels. Although muscarinic receptors are present in the iris, ciliary body, and the retina they have not been isolated from the corneal epithelium.

2.2 Properties of muscarinic agonists

a. Pilocarpine is a direct muscarinic agonist
b. Carbachol is both a direct and an indirect muscarinic agonist
c. These agonists cause miosis and accommodation
d. They decrease intraocular pressure by decreasing production of aqueous
e. Muscarinic agonists decrease intraocular pressure by increasing uveoscleral outflow

Muscarinic agonists may be direct acting (such as pilocarpine) or both direct and indirect acting (for example, carbachol, which inhibits cholinesterase). They cause the triad of miosis (by stimulating the iris sphincter muscle), accommodation (by stimulating the ciliary muscle), and decreased intraocular pressure. The mechanism of the last effect is unknown, but the most widely accepted theory is that these agents produce a passive increase in outflow facility (the scleral spur traction model). Fluorophotometric studies have shown that pilocarpine reduces the intraocular pressure, despite increasing aqueous production and decreasing uveoscleral flow.

2.3 Uses and side effects of cholinergic agonists

> a. Open-angle glaucoma
> b. Esotropias
> c. Reversal of an atropine mydriasis
> d. Diagnosis of Adie's pupils
> e. These agents commonly cause head and brow ache

The main clinical use of cholinergic agonists is in treatment of open angle glaucoma and prophylaxis of closed angle glaucoma, in which treatment halves the incidence of angle closure in the second eye. By decreasing the accommodative effort, cholinergic agonists have been used in the treatment of accommodative squints. Pilocarpine, although it will reverse a phenylephrine mydriasis, will not constrict an atropine mydriasis. Adie's pupils are very sensitive to cholinergic agonists and a solution of pilocarpine of 0.125% will cause a miosis. The most common side effect of these agents is head or brow aches but these normally resolve after 2–3 days.

2.4 Indirect acting muscarinic agonists

> a. Physostigmine acts by phosphorylating cholinesterase
> b. Echothiophate acts by carbamylating cholinesterase
> c. These drugs increase miosis when used in conjunction with pilocarpine
> d. They cause an initial increase in intraocular pressure
> e. Indirect acting agonists reverse an atropine mydriasis

Indirect acting muscarinic agonists (IAMAs) inhibit cholinesterase either by phosphorylation (for example echothioipate), or by carbamylation (for example, physostigmine). Acetylcholine is a more potent miotic than pilocarpine; therefore adding pilocarpine to an IAMA will decrease the miosis. IAMAs produce an initial rise in intraocular pressure, and the eventual hypotensive effect is variable. Some IAMAs will reverse an atropine mydriasis.

2.4 Uses and side effects of IAMAs

a. These drugs lower intraocular pressure
b. They are used in the treatment of esotropias
c. IAMAs are useful to treat lice blepharitis
d. One of the side effects is cataract
e. Their use causes iris nodules

IAMAs such as physostigmine may be used in open angle glaucoma and occasionally as prophylaxis against angle closure glaucoma. However, they are more likely to cause pupil block in the second condition than pilocarpine. They cause less accommodative spasm in esotropias than direct acting agents. Physostigmine will kill *Phthirus pubis* and *Demodex folliculorum*. The risk of cataract with echothiopate is related to dose and duration of treatment and is five times greater than that of pilocarpine. Hyperplasia of the iris pigment epithelium produced by some IAMAs can be prevented by concomitant treatment with phenylephrine.

2.5 Properties of muscarinic antagonists

a. These drugs compete with acetylcholine for receptor sites
b. The order of mydriatic potency in vivo is atropine > cyclopentolate > homatropine > tropicamide
c. They are susceptible to pigment binding
d. Muscarinic antagonists may have a direct α agonist effect
e. Their use decreases the convexity and axial width of the lens

Muscarinic antagonists, naturally occurring or synthetic, act by competing with acetylcholine for receptor sites on the post-synaptic membrane. Their mydriatic effect, which is produced by inhibiting the iris sphincter muscle, is also dependent on drug availability. This explains why tropicamide, which readily penetrates the corneal epithelium, is more effective in vivo than homatropine. Binding of these drugs by pigment accounts for their decreased efficacy and latency of action in pigmented eyes. Atropine may supplement its antimuscarinic action by stimulating α receptors on the dilator muscle. All of these agents will produce cycloplegia by inhibiting the ciliary muscle. This causes thinning and decreased convexity of the lens, reducing the risk of posterior synechiae.

2.6 *Side effects of muscarinic antagonists*

These include:
a. Fever
b. Increase in intraocular pressure
c. Gastrointestinal disturbances
d. Ataxic dysarthria
e. Bradycardia

Minor side-effects associated with muscarinic antagonists are mild fever and skin flushing, which resolve in 24 hours. The intraocular pressure can be raised in several ways, the most obvious of which is precipitation of angle closure; however, these drugs may also decrease aqueous outflow. Pre-testing of patients with open angle glaucoma using 1% cyclopentolate may predict those who will be susceptible to a rise in intraocullar pressure when taking systemic muscarinic antagonists (such as antidepressants and some ulcer medications). Gastrointestinal effects include increased distension and risk of necrotising enterocolitis in neonates. Side-effects on the central nervous system include ataxic dysarthria, cerebellar signs, and an increased risk of seizures. Cardiovascular side effects, if present, tend to be tachyarrhythmias.

3: The adrenergic system

3.1 *Catecholamine receptors in the eye*

> a. α1 Receptors are found in the dilator muscle
> b. α1 Receptors are found in the ciliary muscle
> c. β2 Receptors are found in the central epithelium
> d. β2 Receptors are found in ciliary processes and trabecular meshwork
> e. Dopamine receptors are found in the retina

α1 Receptors are postjunctional ones and are found on the dilator muscle, ciliary muscle, and the sphincter muscle (where they have an inhibitory action). There are no β1 receptors in the eye but β2 receptors are found in the ciliary processes and trabecular meshwork. Dopamine has been isolated from the inner plexiform layer of the retina, where it is thought to be the transmitter in horizontal cells.

3.2 *Properties of catecholamines*

> These drugs:
> a. Decrease aqueous production via α2 and β2 receptors
> b. Increase outflow facility
> c. Decrease uveoscleral flow
> d. Inhibit the iris sphincter muscle
> e. Produce uveal vasoconstriction

The influence of catecholamines on intraocular pressure is controversial. Two possible mechanisms are: (1) a decrease in aqueous production via α2 and β2 receptors is thought to occur by an effect on the non-pigmented ciliary epithelium or by decreasing ciliary blood flow; (2) an increase in outflow facility has been postulated, by direct effects on the trabecular meshwork. Uveoscleral flow is increased indirectly by a decrease in episcleral resistance. Mydriasis occurs by active stimulation of the dilator muscle and active inhibition of the sphincter via α receptors. The vascular tissue of the eye is devoid of β receptors but stimulation of α receptors will cause vasoconstriction.

3.3 *Pharmacology of timolol*

Timolol:
a. Is a relatively selective β1 antagonist
b. Has a duration of action of 6–8 hours
c. Has a greater effect on intraocular pressure than pilocarpine
d. Causes accommodation
e. Is metabolised in the eye

Timolol is a relatively selective β1 antagonist, despite the fact that most receptors in the eye are β2 receptors. This problem is overcome by the aqueous concentrations of timolol, which are 1000 times those required for β2 stimulation. The main effect of the drug is to lower intraocular pressure (which it does more effectively than pilocarpine). Its duration of action of 12–24 hours allows for twice daily administration. Timolol has no effect on the pupillary or ciliary muscles and is metabolised in the liver.

3.4 *Side-effects of ocular β blockers*

a. Depression
b. Bradycardia
c. Wheeze
d. Impotence
e. Superficial punctate keratitis

Ocular β blockers, when absorbed into the circulation, can produce a number of "predictable" side effects. They should be used with caution in patients with heart block and heart failure because of their ability to induce bradyarrhythmias and their negatively inotropic effect. β blockers will also exacerbate bronchospasm in asthmatics or patients with chronic obstructive airways disease. However, new drugs such as betaxolol, which is a selective β1 antagonist, will produce fewer respiratory side effects. Impotence and depression have also been reported, as has superficial punctate keratitis.

3.5 *Properties of adrenaline*

This drug:
a. Stimulates α receptors only
b. Decreases intraocular pressure
c. Causes mydriasis with cycloplegia
d. Causes endothelial cell toxicity
e. Causes macular oedema in aphakic eyes

Adrenaline is both an α and a β agonist. It is known to produce a decrease in intraocular pressure, the magnitude of which is increased when it is used concomitantly with a β blocker. It produces a weak mydriasis without cycloplegia, does not pass readily through the cornea and may cause endothelial toxicity. The risk of macular oedema secondary to topical treatment (which usually resolves when treatment is discontinued) is increased in the aphakic patient.

3.6 *Medications that affect the adrenergic system*

a. Hydroxyamphetamine increases catecholamine release from nerve terminals
b. Cocaine increases catecholamine reuptake
c. Phenylephrine is an α antagonist
d. Phenylephrine may be useful in patients with uveitis
e. Guanethidine may be used to treat lid retraction

Hydroxyamphetamine increases noradrenaline release from nerve terminals and will therefore cause a preganglionic Horner's pupil to dilate. Cocaine inhibits noradrenaline reuptake and will not produce mydriasis in Horner's syndrome, irrespective of its aetiology. Phenylephrine is an α agonist that is useful for breaking posterior synechiae. Guanethidine, which prevents noradrenaline release, has been used topically to treat small degrees of lid retraction by inhibiting contraction of Müller's muscle.

4: Hyperosmotic agents and carbonic anhydrase inhibitors

4.1 *Mannitol*

This agent:
a. Crosses the blood aqueous barrier
b. Causes loss of fluid from the eye by diffusion
c. Should be administered intravenously
d. Is excreted 90% unchanged by the kidneys
e. May have an additional effect on intraocular pressure via optic nerve efferents

Mannitol, like all hyperosmolar agents, does not cross the blood aqueous barrier. It should be given intravenously over a 20–40 minute period and removes water from the eye by osmosis, not diffusion. It is excreted 90% unchanged by the kidneys and therefore should be used with caution in those with compromised renal function because of side effects such as fluid retention and pulmonary oedema. Experimentally, small concentrations of mannitol which do not produce a measurable rise in plasma osmolarity have been found to decrease intraocular pressure. This action is thought to be secondary to hypothalamic efferents travelling in the optic nerve.

4.2 *Glycerol*

a. Glycerol is rapidly absorbed from the gastrointestinal tract
b. It penetrates the inflamed eye better than the non-inflamed eye
c. Hyperosmotic coma is a side effect
d. Ketoacidosis is a side effect
e. Hypoglycaemic coma is a side effect

Glycerol is administered orally and is rapidly absorbed from the gastrointestinal tract. Unlike mannitol, glycerol penetrates more rapidly into the inflamed eye. The average dose of glycerol has a calorific load of 330 calories, which in the diabetic may cause hyperglycaemia, hyperosmotic coma and diabetic ketoacidosis.

4.3 Carbonic anhydrase

a. Carbonic anhydrase catalyses the irreversible reaction $H^+ + HCO_3^- \rightarrow H_2CO_3$
b. It is found in cells of the proximal renal tubules
c. Carbonic anhydrase is found in red blood cells
d. It is found in the pigmented ciliary epithelium
e. The action of this enzyme lowers intraocular pressure

Carbonic anhydrase catalyses the reversible reaction $H^+ + HCO_3^- \leftrightarrow H_2CO_3$. Its bicarbonated form is the body's main buffering agent, playing a vital role in acid–base regulation, and is found in proximal tubule cells (which produce bicarbonate to buffer pH changes in the urine). Carbonic anydrase in red blood cells will catalyse the reaction $CO_2 + H_2O \leftrightarrow H_2CO_3$. The bicarbonate produced dissociates to give H^+ ions (buffered by haemoglobin) and HCO_3^- ions (which diffuse into the plasma). In the non-pigmentary ciliary epithelium, this enzyme stimulates aqueous production, either by increasing bicarbonate availability for cotransport with sodium, or by increasing H^+ concentrations at the inner membrane for sodium transport.

4.4 Uses and side effects of acetazolamide

Acetazolamide:
a. Decreases intraocular pressure
b. May be administered topically
c. Causes parasthesiae
d. Causes depression
e. Causes gastrointestinal upset

Acetazolamide is a carbonic anhydrase inhibitor. It may be administered orally or intravenously. It can produce a marked and rapid decrease in the intraocular pressure but has a number of well documented side effects such as parasthesiae, depression, and gastrointestinal upset. Use of acetazolamide is contraindicated in patients with severe renal impairment.

5: Corticosteroids

5.1 *Anti-inflammatory actions of corticosteroids*

These drugs:
a. Are thought to stabilise lysosomal membranes
b. Increase vascular permeability
c. Increase arteriolar tone
d. Increase adherence of polymorphonucleocytes
e. Inhibit migration of macróphages

Corticosteroids act to modify the body's response to a noxious stimulus. Acute inflammation is characterised by a vascular phase (characterised by increased capillary permeability and dilatation) followed by a cellular phase in which lysosomal release increases the adherence and migration of polymorphs (and macrophages) from the circulation. Corticosteroids are thought to inhibit all these stages of the inflammatory process, but there is no evidence to show how glucocorticoids stabilise lysosomal membranes. New experiments, which show that vitamin E stabilises lysosomal membranes without having any anti-inflammatory effect, cast doubt on this theory.

5.2 Effects of corticosteroids on hypersensitivity, humoral and cell mediated immunity

> a. The effect on T cells is greater than that on B cells
> b. B cells are most sensitive to steroids immediately after antigen presentation
> c. Steroids modify type II and III hypersensitivity reactions
> d. Steroids inhibit histidine decarboxylase and multiplication of eosinophils
> e. Steroids decrease graft versus host reactions

Glucocorticoids modify both humoral and cell mediated immunity by inhibiting B and T lymphocytes respectively. The B cells are most sensitive to corticosteroids immediately after their antigen presentation phase, and type II and type III hypersensitivity reactions can be dampened by decreased antibody production. Type I ·hypersensitivity reactions are lessened because corticosteroids reduce histamine production (by inhibiting histidine decarboxylase) and eosinophil multiplication. Graft versus host reactions are also decreased by administration of steroids because these drugs inhibit T cell mediated macrophages.

5.3 Ocular side effects of systemic corticosteroid therapy

> These include:
> a. Nuclear cataracts
> b. Ptosis
> c. Macular oedema
> d. Mydriasis
> e. Cycloplegia

The most common ocular side effect of systemic corticosteroid treatment is posterior subcapsular cataract. This risk is compounded in conditions (such as rheumatoid arthritis) which themselves predispose to cataract formation. Mild ptosis and mydriasis have also been reported.

5.4 *Side effects of ocular treatment with corticosteroids*

a. Superficial punctate keratitis
b. Disruption of the hypothalamic/pituitary axis
c. Cataracts
d. Scleral melting
e. Contact conjunctivitis/dermatitis

Apart from the obvious side effects (such as HSV dendritic keratitis) corticosteroids used for inappropriate conditions cause superficial punctate keratitis, cataracts and scleral melting. The ingredients of steroid preparations other than the glucocorticoids themselves may also cause an allergic conjunctivitis and/or dermatitis.

5.5 *Corticosteroids and raised intraocular pressure*

a. Few of the general population (6%) are "high" steroid responders
b. Half of the patients with open angle glaucoma are "high" responders
c. The risk of a "high" response to steroids is increased with non-proliferative diabetic retinopathy
d. The risk of a "high" response is increased in hypermetropia
e. Intraocular pressure may be raised by goniocyte swelling in the trabecular meshwork

A patient is said to be a "high" steroid responder if, after a 4 week course of dexamethasone, their intraocular pressure is <30 mmHg (pretreatment pressure <20 mmHg). In the general population 6% of people fall into this category but 90% of patients with open angle glaucoma are "high" responders. Non-proliferative diabetic retinopathy and high myopia also shows an increased incidence of "high" responders. It has been suggested that corticosteroids cause preliminary polymerisation of the mucopolysaccharides in goniocytes, causing them to swell with water and block the drainage angles.

6: Ocular anaesthetics

6.1 *Local anaesthetic agents*

a. These are weak acids
b. They are biphasic
c. Block changes in the sodium permeability of axonal membranes
d. The action is more rapid in myelinated nerves
e. Local anaesthetics are metabolised in the plasma and liver

Local anaesthetics consist of three major parts: a lipophilic aromatic residue is linked to an intermediate aliphatic chain by an ester or amide bond, which is joined to a secondary or tertiary amine. They are weak bases—the charged form binds to the receptor site to prevent sodium influx across axonal membranes. Local anaesthetics can enter myelinated nerves only at the nodes of Ranvier so their rate of action here is considerably slower than in unmyelinated nerves. Most of these drugs are metabolised in the liver or in the plasma.

6.2 *Uses and side effects of topical agents*

Topical anaesthetics:
a. Produce analgesia for approximately 12–20 minutes
b. May have antimicrobial effects
c. Are suitable for systemic use
d. Inhibit epithelial mitoses and migration
e. Cause epithelial loosening and erosions

Four topical anaesthetics are now in common use: cocaine, proparacaine, tetracaine, and benoxinate cause analgesia lasting 10–20 minutes, which takes effect in seconds. Tetracaine and benoxinate have been shown to inhibit growth of some staphylococci, pseudomonas and candida species incubated in 24 hour cultures. Topical anaesthetics are extremely toxic and should never be administered systemically. Side effects are more common with cocaine, and include toxic effects on the metabolism and ultrastructure of epithelial cells (causing erosions), and inhibition of mitoses and migration.

7: Antimitotic and immunosuppressive chemotherapy

7.1 *Properties of azathioprine*

a. Azathioprine is a pyrimidine analogue
b. It is more toxic than mercaptopurine
c. It may cause thrombocytopaenia
d. Azathioprine may cause leukopenia
e. This drug may cause gastrointestinal upset

Azathioprine is a purine analogue which slowly releases mercaptopurine after it is administered, reducing the toxic effects of mercaptopurine. It has been used for a number of ophthalmic conditions such as Graves' disease, scleritis and uveitis secondary to rheumatoid arthritis, herpes zoster ophthalmicus, and sympathetic ophthalmia. Azathioprine is commonly used in combination with systemic steroids. Common side effects include thrombocytopenia, leukopenia and gastrointestinal upset.

7.2 *Properties of cyclosporin*

Cyclosporin:
a. Is a fungal metabolite
b. Has antilymphocytic properties
c. May be used in Behçet's disease
d. Is contraindicated in renal failure
e. May cause thrombocytopenia

Cyclosporin is a fungal metabolite whose antilymphocytic properties have been used in a number of ophthalmic diseases. It is commonly used in conjunction with systemic steroids. In the treatment of Behçet's disease cyclosporin causes a number of well recognised side effects such as nephrotoxicity and thrombocytopenia. It is therefore contraindicated in renal failure, and platelet monitoring is advisable.

8: Ocular side effects of systemic medications

8.1 *The following may cause pseudotumour cerebrae*

a. Tetracycline
b. Ethambutol
c. Vitamin A
d. Chloramphenicol
e. Corticosteroids

Tetracycline, vitamin A and systemic corticosteroids may all cause pseudotumour cerebrae, a condition in which the intracranial pressure is raised and the patient presents with symptoms of headaches, nausea, and vomiting with associated papilloedema. Ethambutol and chloramphenicol are causes of optic neuropathy.

8.2 *Corneal deposits may be caused by*

a. Chloroquine
b. Tamoxifen
c. Practolol
d. Amiodarone
e. Thioridazine

Chloroquine may produce corneal epithelial deposits with associated retinal degeneration. Amiodarone produces a characteristic pattern of epithelial deposits, which are reversible on cessation of treatment. Tamoxifen, used in the treatment of breast carcinoma, may also produce corneal deposits which are normally subepithelial. Thioridazine, a phenothiazine type drug, is also known to cause corneal deposits.

8.3 *Cataract may be caused by*

a. Oral hypoglycaemics
b. Phenytoin
c. Glucocorticoids
d. Amiodarone
e. Thioridazine

Oral hypoglycocaemics and glucocorticoids are known to cause posterior subcapsular cataracts. Amiodarone and thioridazine may also produce lens deposits but the only known ocular side effect of phenytoin is nystagmus.

Answers

1.1	b	**3.2**	a, b, d, e	**5.3**	b, d
1.2	a, c, e	**3.3**	a, c	**5.4**	a, c, d, e
1.3	a, b, d	**3.4**	a, b, c, d, e	**5.5**	a, c, e
		3.5	b, d, e		
2.1	a, c	**3.6**	a, d, e	**6.1**	b, c, e
2.2	a, b, c			**6.2**	a, b, d, e
2.3	a, b, d, e	**4.1**	c, d, e		
2.4	d, e	**4.2**	a, b, c, d	**7.1**	c, d, e
2.4	a, b, c, d, e	**4.3**	b, c	**7.2**	a, b, c, d, e
2.5	a, c, d, e	**4.4**	a, c, d, e		
2.6	a, b, c, d			**8.1**	a, c, e
		5.1	a, e	**8.2**	a, b, d, e
3.1	a, b, d, e	**5.2**	a, b, c, d, e	**8.3**	a, c, d, e

Ocular physiology

1: The lacrimal apparatus

1.1 *Lacrimal gland*

> This gland
> a. Is a tubuloacinar gland
> b. Has ducts lined with a squamous epithelium
> c. Receives postganglionic secretomotor fibres from the ciliary ganglion
> d. Develops from neuroectoderm
> e. Contains predominantly serous secretory cells

The lacrimal gland is a tubuloacinar gland derived from surface ectoderm with ducts lined by a low columnar or cuboidal epithelium (often bilayered). The secretory cells in the acini have a predominance of dense granules, suggesting that most are of a serous nature. However, some cells are mucus producing. The postganglionic secretomotor fibres (which arise from the pterygopalatine ganglion) "hitch-hike" on the zygomatico-temporal and lacrimal nerves to the gland.

1.2 *Tear production*

> a. The lacrimal gland is responsible for basal secretion
> b. Wolfring's glands produce more tears than Krause's glands
> c. Trauma to the superior salivatory nucleus decreases reflex tearing
> d. Sympathetic nerves influence tear production
> e. Psychogenic tearing is always bilateral

Basal secretions are produced by the glands of Krause and to a lesser extent by the glands of Wolfring. The lacrimal gland is responsible for reflex tearing and its parasympathetic input arises from the superior salivatory nucleus. Sympathetic nerves may influence lacrimal secretions by altering the blood flow to the gland. Psychogenic tearing is always bilateral.

1.3 *The tear film*

a. The tear film is composed of three layers
b. The main function of the lipid layer is to reduce evaporation of the aqueous layer
c. The mucin layer is 10 μm thick and is hydrophobic
d. The goblet cells have their greatest concentration inferonasally
e. Tear film break-up time is normally approximately 5–10 seconds

The tear film is composed of three layers: a lipid layer (produced predominantly by the tarsal glands) reduces evaporation of the second (aqueous) layer, which is produced by the basal secretions from the glands of Krause and Wolfring. The inner (hydophilic mucin) layer, produced by the goblet cells (whose greatest concentration is inferonasal), is 0·05 μm thick and enables the tear film to spread evenly over the hydrophobic corneal and conjunctival epithelium. The healthy tear film has a break-up time of approximately 10–30 seconds.

1.4 *Tear dynamics*

a. The maximum volume of the conjunctival sac is 30 μl
b. The average tear film volume is 15 μl
c. Tear film turnover time is approximately 18% per minute
d. The volume of a "drop" of topical medication is approximately 50 μl
e. A normal Schirmer's test is approximately 15–25 mm of "wetting" over 5 minutes

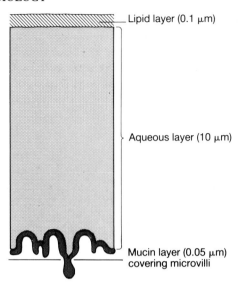

Lipid layer (0.1 μm)

Aqueous layer (10 μm)

Mucin layer (0.05 μm) covering microvilli

Fig 67 The tear film

The maximum volume of the conjunctival sac is 20 μl but the normal tear volume is approximately 6–7 μl because of the effect of blinking. This explains why only 20% of an average drop of medication (approximately 50 μl) is retained in the conjunctival sac, the rest being lost to overflow. A tear turnover rate of 18% per minute compounds poor retention of medication, which means that after 5 minutes only 40% of the medication is present in the conjunctival sac. A normal Schirmer's test would produce 15–25 mm of "wetting" over a period of 5 minutes.

1.5 *Tear biochemistry*

a. The osmolarity of tears is approximately that of normal saline
b. The pH of tears is 7.0
c. The potassium content of tears is 3–5 times that of plasma
d. The chloride content of tears is less than that of plasma
e. The glucose concentration of tears is greater than that of the plasma

The osmolarity of tears is approximately that of normal saline and the pH is 7.4. The potassium concentration is 15–30 mmol/l and the chloride concentration (135 mmol/l) is greater than that of plasma. The tear film supplies the corneal epithelium with glucose—its glucose concentration is therefore less than that of plasma.

1.6 *Protein content of tears*

a. Albumin accounts for 60% of total tear protein
b. IgG and IgA are found in roughly equal concentrations
c. Lysozyme acts in a similar way to penicillin type drugs
d. Lysozyme concentrations decrease with age
e. Enzyme disorders can be diagnosed from tear assays

Albumin accounts for 60% of tear protein. The ratio of IgG to IgA in serum is 7:1—this ratio is 1:1 in the tear film. Lysozyme's protective action is achieved by breakdown of bacterial cell walls and its concentration decreases steadily with age. Many inborn errors of metabolism (such as Hurler's syndrome) can be detected by assays of tears.

2: The eyelids

2.1 *Reflex blinking*

Reflex blinking:
a. May be caused by optical stimulation
b. May be caused by auditory stimulation
c. A corneal reflex is dependent on the fifth and seventh cranial nerves
d. Cortical function is needed for a corneal reflex
e. Is initiated by the pretarsal fibres of orbicularis oculi

Reflex blinking may be caused by optical, auditory or tactile stimuli. Tactile stimulation of the cornea triggers a brain stem reflex via the fifth and seventh cranial nerves and therefore does not require a cortical input. Tumours of the cerebellopontine angle often cause a loss of the corneal reflex before other branches of the fifth nerve are affected. The pretarsal (as opposed to the orbital) fibres of orbicularis oculi initiate the action of reflex blinking.

2.2 Spontaneous blinking

a. Spontaneous blinking is absent until the third month of life
b. Blind people blink spontaneously
c. Frequency is approximately 15 per minute
d. Spontaneous blinking is preceded by relaxation of levator palpebrae superioris
e. Duration is approximately 1–1.5 seconds

Spontaneous blinking is absent until the third month of life and, as it does not require retinal stimulation, is present in blind people. The blink lasts 0.3–0.4 seconds and is preceded by relaxation of levator palpebrae superioris. It is responsible for spreading the tear film over the cornea and conjunctiva and occurs about 15 times each minute.

2.3 Associated eye movements

a. Upward movement of the globe associated with eye closure is known as the pseudo Graefe phenomenon
b. Bell's phenomenon is absent in 10% of normal people
c. Voluntary upward gaze is associated with lid retraction
d. Fibrillary twitching of the eyelids may be due to refractive error
e. The Marcus Gunn syndrome is caused by pterygoid linkage of and levator palpebrae superioris

Bell's phenomenon is the upward movement of the globe associated with eye closure and is absent in 10% of normal people. The Marcus Gunn syndrome (or jaw winking) is caused by levator palpebrae superioris and pterygoid muscle linkage (it is not known whether this is at a cortical or peripheral nerve level). Fibrillary twitching may be caused by refractive errors.

2.4 Effect of drugs on eyelids

a. Guanethidine can be used to decrease width of the palpebral fissure
b. Botulinum toxin inhibits release of acetylcholine from presynaptic terminals
c. Botulinum toxin is used in the treatment of blepharospasm
d. Edrophonium acts as an indirect nicotinic agonist in the Tensilon test
e. The partial ptosis of Horner's syndrome is reversed by topical cocaine

Guanethidine acts by inhibiting release of noradrenaline from nerve terminals (chemical sympathectomy) and will therefore inhibit the action of Müller's muscle, so decreasing palpebral fissure width. The therapeutic action of botulinum toxin in blepharospasm is achieved by inhibiting presynaptic acetylcholine release and decreasing neuromuscular transmission. A Tensilon test (used in the diagnosis of myasthenia gravis) uses the anticholinergic action of edrophonium at neuromuscular junctions, increasing the concentration of acetylcholine at these junctions. Cocaine prevents reuptake of noradrenaline but will enhance sympathetic activity only if there is an intact sympathetic chain to initiate release of the noradrenaline. It will therefore not affect the partial ptosis seen in Horner's syndrome.

3: The cornea

3.1 *Physical properties of the cornea*

a. The refractive power of the anterior corneal surface is 48.8 dioptres
b. The cornea represents 50% of the eye's refractive power
c. The anterior corneal surface is hyperboloid in shape
d. The vertical meridian usually has a shorter radius of curvature than the horizontal meridian
e. The refractive index of the cornea is 1.376

The anterior corneal surface has a refractive power of 48.8 dioptres and the posterior surface − 5.8 dioptres: 43 dioptres in total. This accounts for 70% of the eye's refractive power. The anterior surface is steepest centrally and flattened peripherally, giving it a hyperboloidal shape. The vertical meridian has the shorter radius of curvature and hence an increased refractive power in 95% of eyes. The refractive index of the cornea is 1.376.

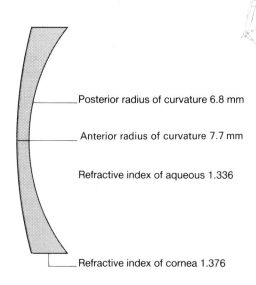

Posterior radius of curvature 6.8 mm

Anterior radius of curvature 7.7 mm

Refractive index of aqueous 1.336

Refractive index of cornea 1.376

Fig 68 Physical properties of the cornea

3.2 *Corneal structure*

a. The cornea consists of five layers
b. Bowman's membrane is capable of regeneration
c. Descemet's membrane is capable of regeneration
d. Bowman's membrane is more resistant to solvent flow than Descemet's membrane
e. Endothelial cells are joined by zonula adherens and zonula occludens

The cornea is made up of five layers. The epithelium (the most superficial layer) is separated from the stroma by Bowman's membrane. Both Bowman's and Descemet's membranes (adjacent to Bowman's membrane) are 10 μm thick, but Descemet's membrane is able to regenerate and is more resistant to the flow of solvent. The deepest layer is the endothelium: tight junctions between adjacent endothelial cells are essential for controlling corneal hydration.

3.3 *Biochemistry of the cornea*

a. Water makes up 60% of stromal weight
b. Glycosaminoglycans are bound to stromal collagen
c. Keratan sulphate is the most common glycosaminoglycan in the cornea
d. The epithelium is rich in glycolytic and Krebs' cycle enzymes
e. Oxygen consumption by the endothelium is 12 times that of the stroma

The stroma consists of water (80%), glycosaminoglycans (such as keratan and chondroitin sulphate), and mucopolysaccharides bind collagen and account for 5% of the dry weight. The stroma has a very low cell count per unit volume, which explains why corneal oxygen consumption is eight times lower than that of the epithelium and 12 times lower than that of the endothelium, both of which are rich in glycolytic and Krebs' cycle enzymes.

3.4 *Electrolyte and glucose content of corneal layers*

a. The epithelial potassium concentration is approximately 140 mmol/l
b. The epithelial sodium concentration is approximately 70 mmol/l
c. The glucose needs of the epithelium are supplied by the aqueous
d. The stromal potassium concentration is half that of the epithelium
e. Stromal electroneutrality is maintained by anionic glycosaminoglycans

A sodium–potassium ATPase pump in the corneal epithelium ensures that potassium concentrations are kept high and sodium concentrations relatively low. The glucose needs of the epithelium are supplied by the tear film and those of the endothelium by the aqueous. Stromal potassium is approximately 20 mmol/l (seven times longer than that of the epithelium) and its low chloride concentration (110 mmol/l) is compensated for by anionic glycosaminoglycans which maintain electroneutrality.

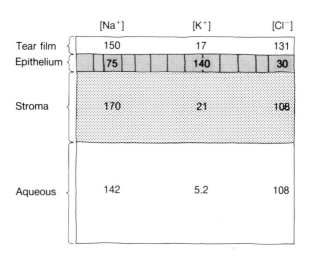

Fig 69 Electrolyte concentrations (mmol/l) of the tear film, cornea and aqueous

3.5 *Corneal dehydration*

a. Dehydration of the cornea is dependent on an intact endothelium
b. Epithelial trauma causes marked and persistent corneal swelling
c. Ouabain causes corneal swelling
d. Intraocular pressure may influence corneal hydration
e. Tear film tonicity may influence corneal hydration

In order for the cornea to dehydrate an intact corneal endothelium and epithelium are essential. Epithelial trauma will cause only a mild and transient oedema. Ouabain inhibits the sodium–potassium ATPase essential for corneal dehydration. Intraocular pressure, if above 50 mmHg, will cause corneal oedema. Application of glycerin to the tear film increases its osmolarity and causes water to be drawn from the cornea, so decreasing oedema.

3.6 *Corneal transparency*

a. Light scattering is eliminated by mutual interference (Maurice's theory)
b. Fluid overload is the only cause for loss of transparency
c. A regular stromal collagen lattice is essential for transparency
d. Regional fluctuations in the corneal refractive index may explain destructive interference patterns
e. Collagen fibres and glycosaminoglycans from micelles with water

Several theories have been put forward to account for corneal transparency (or the lack of it). Maurice stated that the light scattering is eliminated by mutual interference—which requires a regular collagen lattice. Such a lattice is maintained by the formation of micelles between stromal water, collagen, and glycosaminoglycans. Sharks, however, do not have a regular lattice but do have transparent corneas. Goldmann concluded the destructive interference patterns may be explained by fluctuations in refractive index. Deformity of the corneal lattice caused by increased intraocular pressure (not necessarily an increased water content) also reduces transparency of the cornea.

3.7 *The avascular cornea*

a. It is normal to find vessels 1 mm from the limbus
b. Vascularisation is caused by swelling
c. Vitamin A deficiency causes vascularisation
d. Angiogenic inhibitory factors may be involved
e. Vascularisation increases graft survival

Corneal vascularisation was initially thought to be caused by corneal swelling. However, hydrops cornea does not cause vascularisation and vitamin A deficiency produces marked vascularisation with no swelling. Angiogenic inhibitory factors have been implicated but never isolated. Vascularisation means that the cornea loses its immunologically "privileged" site and graft survival is decreased.

3.8 *Corneal wounds*

a. Epithelial mitoses occur at the edge of the wound
b. Epithelial migration is simulated by fibronectin
c. Chalones inhibit cell division
d. Adrenaline decreases epithelial mitosis
e. Large doses of ultraviolet light increase epithelial mitoses

The epithelial cells at the corneal limbus divide, and under the influence of fibronectin and decreasing concentrations of chalones (secondary to epithelial cell loss) migrate to repair the defect. Adrenaline is known to inhibit epithelial mitosis, as does large doses of ultraviolet light. Small doses of ultraviolet light are thought to promote healing.

3.9 *Corneal sensation*

---

a. Pain receptors are found in the stroma
b. Cold receptors are found in the epithelium
c. Heat receptors are found in the epithelium
d. Pain from the cornea is well localised
e. Pain impulses travel in "c" nerve fibres

Pain receptors are found in the epithelium, not the stroma. Cold receptors are found in the deeper layers of the epithelium but there is no evidence of heat receptors in the cornea. The density of pain receptors is very high in the cornea and therefore pain sensation is well localised, unlike pain sensation caused by noxious stimulation of the iris, which has a less dense innervation. This information is conveyed in Aδ fast pain fibres.

4: The aqueous and intraocular pressure

4.1 *Ciliary epithelium*

---

a. The ciliary epithelium has two layers derived from neuroectoderm
b. The outer layer is continuous with the retinal pigment epithelium
c. The inner layer is rich in mitochondria, rough endoplasmic reticulum and golgi apparatus
d. The cells of the bilayered epithelium lie base to base
e. The inner and outer layers are joined by tight junctions

The ciliary epithelium is a bilayered structure derived from the neuroectoderm of the optic vesicle. The inner layer is rich in mitochondria, rough endoplasmic reticulum and golgi apparatus. It is a continuation of the neural layer of the retina. The outer pigmented layer is a continuation of the retinal pigment epithelial layer. Tight junctions exist between adjacent cells in the inner layer, but not between the cells of the different layers or between cells of the outer layer. The outer layer cells are connected by gap junctions.

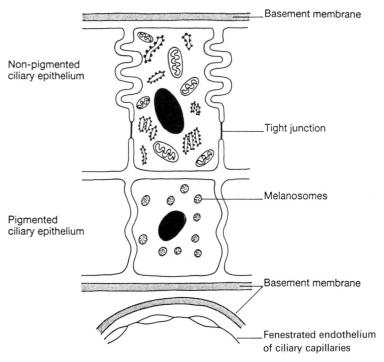

Basement membrane

Non-pigmented
ciliary epithelium

Tight junction

Melanosomes

Pigmented
ciliary epithelium

Basement membrane

Fenestrated endothelium
of ciliary capillaries

Fig 70 The ciliary epithelium

4.2 Components of the blood aqueous barrier

a. Non-fenestrated ciliary capillaries
b. Tight junctions between non-pigmented ciliary epithelial cells
c. Non-fenestrated iris vessels
d. Tight junctions between pigmented ciliary epithelial cells
e. Tight junctions between endothelial cells of iris vessels

The blood aqueous barrier in the posterior chamber is maintained because the tight junctions between the inner non-pigmented epithelial cells prevent exudate from the fenestrated ciliary capillaries reaching the aqueous. The iris has no protective epithelial barrier and relies on non-fenestrated vessels to maintain the blood aqueous barrier. However, the endothelial cells of these vessels are not joined by tight junctions and in inflammatory conditions they become "leaky," causing an aqueous flare.

4.3 Causes of disruption of the blood aqueous barrier

a. Paracentesis
b. Irin (prostaglandins E and F)
c. Intracarotid injection of hyperosmolar agents
d. Laser trabeculoplasty
e. Prostaglandins

All of the above may destroy the blood aqueous barrier. Irin consists of prostaglandins E and F and causes breakdown of the tight junctions in the non-pigmented epithelium. Hyperosmolar agents may cause the pigmented and non-pigmented epithelial layers to separate.

4.4 Formation of aqueous humour

a. Ouabain decreases production by less than 20%
b. Ultrafiltration is the major factor in aqueous production
c. Osmosis plays a small role
d. Adenylate cyclase and carbonic anhydrase may be involved
e. Production is approximately 2.5 ml/min

The major factor (approximately 70%) involved in aqueous production is "active secretion" via the sodium–potassium ATPase pump. This is situated in the clefts of the non-pigmented epithelium, acts independently of intraocular pressure, and is inhibited by ouabain. Ultrafiltration is thought to play a relatively minor role in aqueous production, as is osmosis. Aqueous production is thought to be controlled by cyclic AMP which is regulated by adrenylate cyclase. Carbonic anhydrase is found in the ciliary processes, and by altering HCO_3^- : H^+ ratios will affect aqueous production. Aqueous production is approximately 2.5 μl/min.

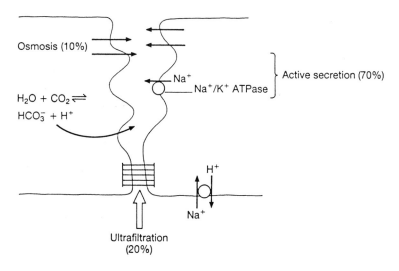

Fig 71 **Aqueous production by the non-pigmented epithelium**

4.5 *Functions of the aqueous*

a. The aqueous supplies amino acids to the lens
b. It supplies glucose to the corneal epithelium
c. The aqueous maintains intraocular pressure
d. The aqueous is a transparent conducting medium
e. It is responsible for focusing light on the retina

The main functions of the aqueous are
(1) to supply nutrition to the lens, corneal endothelium, and stroma—but not to the epithelium which relies on tears for its nutrition;
(2) to maintain intraocular pressure;
(3) to remain transparent

4.6 Composition of the aqueous

> a. The sodium content is similar to that of the corneal epithelium
> b. The potassium content is approximately 4 mmol/l
> c. The glucose content is approximately 80% that of plasma
> d. The lactate concentration is greater than that of the plasma
> e. Aqueous has relatively low ascorbic acid content

The electrolyte composition of aqueous is similar to that of the plasma. The concentration of sodium (140 mmol/l) is twice that of the corneal epithelium; the potassium concentration is approximately 4 mmol/l. Owing to its nutritional function, aqueous glucose concentration is 80% of that of plasma. Lactate produced by the cornea and lens is excreted into the aqueous, increasing its levels relative to plasma. The ascorbic acid concentration in the aqueous is high. Several roles for ascorbic acid have been postulated, including absorption of ultraviolet light and an action as an antioxidant.

4.7 Protein content of the aqueous

> a. The protein content of the aqueous is half that of plasma
> b. There is a high albumin:globulin ratio
> c. All immunoglobulins are usually detectable
> d. Plasminogen is present
> e. Increases with disruption of the blood aqueous barrier

The protein content of the aqueous is 1/90th that of plasma because of the blood aqueous barrier; any disruption of this barrier will increase protein influx. The albumin:globulin ratio is high, and IgG is the only globulin detectable in the aqueous. Plasminogen and its proactivator are present, but none of their inhibitors or other clotting factors are detectable in the aqueous.

211

4.8 *Dynamics of the aqueous*

> a. Outflow is usually described by two pathways
> b. Uveoscleral flow is approximately 0.3 µl per minute
> c. Trabecular outflow is dependent on the intraocular and episcleral pressures
> d. Uveoscleral flow is not affected by the intraocular pressure
> e. Aqueous inflow is constant over a wide range of intraocular pressure

Aqueous outflow is usually described by two separate pathways. Most of the flow is through the trabecular meshwork and canal of Schlemm, dependent on the intraocular and episcleral venous pressures. Uveoscleral outflow is approximately 0.3 µl/min and is surprisingly independent of intraocular pressure changes. Aqueous production will remain constant until intraocular pressures are raised to 50 mmHg and over.

4.9 *Outflow mechanics*

> a. The flow in a vessel is proportional to the fourth power of the radius of that vessel
> b. Aqueous flow is proportional to resistance in the "vessel" over the pressure difference along it
> c. The capacitance and resistance are inversely related
> d. The trabecular outflow resistance changes with increasing intraocular pressure
> e. Brubaker's correction is related to aqueous outflow

The Poiseuille Hagen Formula states that the resistance to blood flow in a vessel is inversely proportional to the fourth power of its radius, and hence flow in that vessel is directly proportional to the fourth power of the radius.

$$R = 8\eta L/\pi r^4$$

where: R = resistance; η = viscosity; L = length of vessel; r = radius of vessel

The flow of aqueous through the trabecular meshwork (I) will depend on the pressure difference between the intraocular pressure and the episcleral venous pressure (V) divided by the resistance of the trabecular meshwork (R)—a simple adaptation of Ohm's law ($V = IR$; $I = V/R$). The capacitance is the inverse of the resistance ($I = VC$) and the trabecular meshwork capacitance is seen to decrease as intraocular pressure rises. Brubaker's correction allows for this when calculating aqueous outflow.

4.10 Drainage of the trabecular meshwork

a. Drainage is predominantly by ultrafiltration
b. Tight junctions exist between endothelial cells of Schlemm's canal
c. Vacuole formation is involved in aqueous drainage
d. Parasympathetic stimulation decreases aqueous outflow
e. Scotopic conditions are likely to worsen aqueous outflow

Drainage through Schlemm's canal (which is lined by endothelial cells joined by tight junctions) is the main route of aqueous outflow. Aqueous is thought to be transported in large vacuoles, which pass through the endothelial cells lining the meshwork. When the ciliary muscle contracts secondary to parasympathetic stimulation, the oblique fibres of the trabecular meshwork are stretched. This in turn increases the size of Schlemm's canal and aids outflow. Conversely, in scotopic conditions the pupil dilates and the angle narrows, increasing outflow resistance.

4.11 *Intraocular pressure*

a. Intraocular pressure always exhibits a diurnal rhythm
b. It has a seasonal variation
c. Pressure is generally higher in males
d. The diurnal variation is less in glaucomatous eyes
e. Intraocular pressure is increased by the Valsalva manoeuvre

In most people intraocular pressure exhibits a diurnal rhythm, the peaks and troughs of which vary between individuals. This variation is exaggerated in glaucomatous eyes. The usual peak occurs late in the morning (12.00–13.00), and the trough early in the morning (03.00–04.00). Statistically, intraocular pressure is higher in the winter and lower in the summer. There is little difference between males and females until the age of 40, when the intraocular pressure becomes generally higher in women. The Valsalva manoeuvre will increase venous pressure generally, and therefore episcleral venous pressure will also rise. This will cause a transient increase in intraocular pressure.

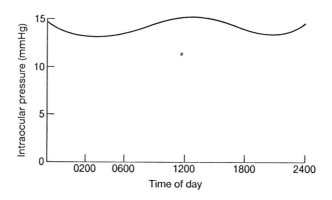

Fig 72 Diurnal variation of intraocular pressure

4.12 *Intraocular pressure*

a. Mean value in the population is 15–16 mmHg
b. Intraocular pressure decreases with age
c. During induction of anaesthesia intraocular pressure may rise
d. Pressure may increase in extreme positions of gaze
e. When sleeping the intraocular pressure decreases

The intraocular pressure exhibits a normal distribution in the population, and has a mean value of approximately 12–14 mmHg. Intraocular pressure tends to increase with age, the reasons for which are thought to be multifactorial. Both sleep and general anaesthesia produce a prompt decrease in intraocular pressure secondary to a loss of intraocular muscle tone. However, agents such as suxamethonium can produce a transient but marked rise in intraocular pressure, which is especially undesirable in perforating injuries. The rise in intraocular pressure in extremes of gaze varies between individuals and the direction of gaze.

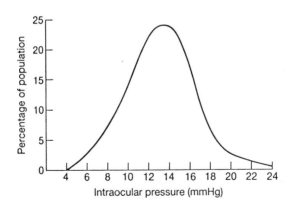

Fig 73 Distribution of intraocular pressure

5: **The lens**

5.1 *Functions*

The lens is responsible for:
a. Accommodation
b. Maintenance of transparency
c. Filtering infrared light
d. The main refractive power of the eye
e. Forming part of the blood aqueous barrier

The lens accounts for approximately 30% of the refractive power of the eye and is capable of changing shape so that images of objects at varying distances from the eye may be focused on the retina—this is known as accommodation. To carry out these functions, the lens must remain transparent. The lens will absorb light at the blue end of the visual spectrum but does not form part of the blood aqueous barrier.

5.2 *Optics*

a. The anterior radius of curvature is 6 mm
b. The posterior radius of curvature is 10 mm
c. The refractive index of the nucleus is greater than that of the cortex
d. The accommodative power is approximately 14 dioptres in a 10 year old
e. Lens size increases throughout life

The anterior curvature of the lens is 10 mm and that of the posterior surface 6 mm. However, these values will change with age because the cells of the equatorial lens epithelium continue to divide throughout life, increasing the size of the lens. The refractive index of the lens nucleus is approximately 1.41, greater than that of the lens cortex, which is 1.39. The accommodative power of the lens of a 10 year old is approximately 14 dioptres—this decreases to 10 dioptres by the age of 20.

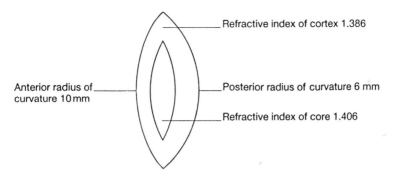

Fig 74 Physical properties of the lens

5.3 *Biochemistry*

> a. Sodium is actively transported into the lens
> b. Chloride passively diffuses into the lens
> c. The potassium content of the lens is five times that of the aqueous
> d. The glucose content is approximately one-sixth of that of the aqueous
> e. Amino acids are actively transported into the lens

The sodium–potassium ATPase pump in the lens epithelium maintains a sodium concentration of approximately 20 mmol/l and a potassium concentration of 125 mmol/l (25 times that of the aqueous). Chloride ions follow an electrochemical gradient and passively diffuse into the lens. Glucose is derived from the aqueous, as are amino acids which are actively transported across the epithelium.

5.4 *Lens proteins*

> a. Protein accounts for 33% of the lens weight
> b. Insoluble proteins account for 85% of lens proteins
> c. β Crystallin is the most common soluble protein
> d. α Crystallin is found predominantly in the cortex
> e. Lens proteins make up the anion gap

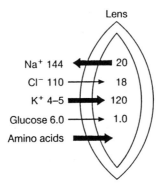

Fig 75 Chemical transport between the lens and aqueous. ➡ **Active transport;** → **diffusion. All concentrations are in mmol/l**

The protein content of the lens is higher than in any other body tissue (33% of lens weight). Soluble proteins such as α, β, and γ crystallins make up 85% of the total protein content. β Crystallin accounts for 50% of these soluble proteins; α crystallin is predominantly found in the cortex. Leakage of these proteins from mature cataracts can precipitate a phacoanaphylactic uveitis and/or glaucoma. The anion gap formed by the relatively low chloride and bicarbonate content of the lens is redressed by its high protein content.

5.5 *Metabolism of the lens*

a. The cholesterol:phospholipid ratio is the highest of any tissue
b. Glycolysis is responsible for 80% of lens energy production
c. The hexosemonophosphate shunt utilises 15% of glucose in the lens
d. Hexokinase becomes saturated in hyperglycaemia
e. Excess sorbitol accumulation in the diabetic lens is the major factor in diabetic cataractogenesis

Lipids account for 5% of the dry weight of the lens (cholesterol approximately 50%, phospholipid 45%, glycosphingolipids 5%) and the cholesterol:phospholipid ratio is higher than in any other tissue. Glycolysis utilises 80% of the lens glucose but does not produce a correspondingly high percentage of the ATP output as glycolysis will produce a net gain of only 2 ATP for every glucose molecule. The hexosemonophosphate shunt utilises 15% of lens glucose, a relatively high percentage compared with other tissues. In hyperglycaemic states hexokinase becomes saturated and glucose is channelled into the sorbitol pathway, increasing sorbitol production. A theory of diabetic cataract formation, widely quoted in ophthalmic texts, is that this high sorbitol concentration draws water into the lens by osmosis, resulting in vacuolisation and eventually cataract formation. However, sorbitol in the lens is rapidly converted to fructose, which diffuses into the aqueous before any osmotic gradient can be established! Cataract formation in the diabetic is primarily caused by glycosylation of lens proteins with the subsequent disruption of the sodium–potassium ATPase pump.

5.6 *Glutathione*

a. Glutathione is a five amino acid polypeptide
b. Approximately 90% of glutathione is in the oxidized form
c. Glutathione is involved in detoxification of free radicals
d. Glutathione helps maintain the integrity of lens proteins by preventing protein cross linkage formation
e. A reduction of lens glutathione is a consistent finding in senile cataracts

Glutathione (a three amino acid polypeptide) is found in high concentrations in the lens. Mostly (93%) it is found in its reduced form (GSH), and is maintained thus by the NADPH produced by the hexosemonophosphate shunt. Glutathione is vital for the maintenance of lens transparency in maintaining the integrity of lens proteins of the sodium–potassium ATPase pump (by preventing protein cross linkages and maintaining essential thiols). A reduction of lens GSH is a consistent finding in senile and all tested experimental cataracts. Glutathione peroxidase is involved in the detoxification of hydrogen peroxide, some of which is formed from O_2^- radicals.

5.7 *Chemical changes in cataractogenesis*

These may include:
a. Decreased glutathione levels
b. Increased potassium and amino acid efflux
c. Disulphide bond formation between lens proteins
d. Sorbitol formation
e. Increased galactilol formation

Decreased glutathione concentrations will lead to malfunction of the sodium membrane pump, causing an efflux of potassium and amino acids and an influx of sodium and water. Such malfunction is often a result of disulphide linkages forming between lens proteins. The increased sorbitol production seen in diabetes and increased galactilol production resulting from galactosaemia both predispose to cataract formation.

6: Accommodation

6.1 *Lenticular changes in accommodation*

a. The anterior pole of the lens moves forward
b. Axial width of the lens increases
c. There is no change in tension of the lens capsule
d. The lens always moves inferiorly
e. There is a physiological lentoconus

In accommodating for near vision the circular ciliary muscle contracts, decreasing the tension in the zonular fibres, and allowing the lens capsule to contract and change the shape of the lens. The anterior pole moves anteriorly, the axial width increases and the equatorial diameter of the lens decreases. The lens will move in the direction of gravity as the zonule slackens: this will only be inferiorly if the person is upright. The anterior curvature was considered to increase to a greater extent than the posterior curvature, causing a physiological lentoconus, but although this appears to be true when using the slitlamp it is probably an artefact of corneal refraction.

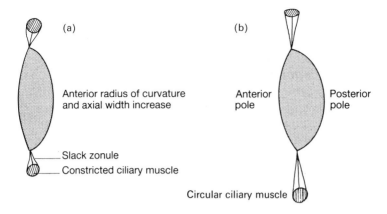

Fig 76 Lenticular changes during accommodation: (a) accommodating eye; (b) related eye

6.2 *The near triad*

a. Pupillary dilatation, accommodation and convergence make up the triad
b. The near triad is a true reflex
c. Accommodation occurs first
d. The pupillary response is slower than the response to light
e. Blur is the main stimulus to accommodation

The near triad consists of convergence, accommodation and pupillary constriction (not dilatation). It is not a true reflex but is a synkineisis—no component of the triad depends on the other two for its appearance, so that if accommodation is prevented (using a convex lens) and the eye converges to the near point the pupil will still constrict. Accommodation is the slowest reaction of the triad, taking between 0.56 s (near to far) and 0.64 s (far to near). The main stimulus for accommodation is image blur. The pupillary response is approximately 0.26–0.2 s; this is slower than the reaction to light.

OCULAR PHYSIOLOGY

6.3 *Lens capsule*

> a. The capsule is of uniform thickness
> b. Capsular changes are active
> c. Intralenticular pressure is greatest in the unaccommodated state
> d. The lens capsule is more fragile in the diabetic
> e. Capsular antigens are similar to those found in glomerular basement membranes

The lens capsule is not uniformly thick, the capsule over the anterior and posterior poles being slightly thinner than the equatorial capsule. The capsule is inherently elastic and changes in its shape (which are passive) occur because of increased pressure within the lens in the unaccommodated state. The capsule is more fragile in the diabetic lens. Capsular antigens are similar to those found in glomerular basement membranes.

6.4 *Properties of zonular fibres*

> a. Zonular fibres connect the ciliary process to the lens
> b. Zonular fibres are uncrossed
> c. Zonular fibres connect the pars plana to the vitreous
> d. Zonular fibres are acellular and have no metabolism
> e. Cystine makes up approximately 7% of fibre weight

Zonular fibres arise from the ciliary body and may be divided into two groups: those that pass from the ciliary processes to the lens, most of which attach to the anterior or posterior lens capsule rather than the equator and do not seem to cross each other; and zonular fibres that either form a meshwork across the ciliary body, or extend from the pars plana to the vitreous body to form part of the vitreous base. Both types are acellular and have a cystine concentration of approximately 7%. This explains why lens dislocation is a common feature of homocystinuria.

6.5 *Properties of the ciliary muscle*

a. This is a striated muscle
b. The ciliary muscle is stimulated by muscarinic antagonists
c. Contraction of the ciliary muscle accommodation
d. The ciliary muscle is attached to the scleral spur
e. This muscle is composed solely of longitudinal fibres

The ciliary muscle is a smooth muscle consisting predominantly of longitudinal fibres that bend anteriorly to form a circle. Other longitudinal fibres pass to the anterior choroid and oblique fibres pass to the scleral spur. When stimulated by muscarinic agonists the ciliary muscle produces accommodation, and pulls the choroid anteriorly—the increased traction on the trabecular fibres via the scleral spur aids aqueous outflow.

6.6 *Changes in accommodative power*

a. Accommodation is well developed by 2 months
b. The accommodative power for a 20 year old is approximately 10 dioptres
c. The accommodative power of a 2 year old is approximately 20 dioptres
d. Accommodation is absent by the age of 60
e. Accommodative loss is seen in Adie's syndrome

Accommodation begins to develop at the age of 2 months and is well developed by the eighth month of life. The accommodative power of a 2 year old lens is approximately 20 dioptres. By the age of 20 years this has decreased to 10 dioptres, and at 60 years of age accommodation is no longer possible. In Adie's syndrome damage to the ciliary ganglion causes loss of accommodation and explains the initial symptom, which is blurring of vision.

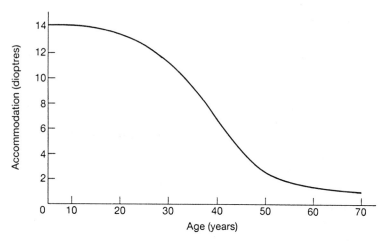

Fig 77 Changes in accommodative power with age

7: The vitreous

7.1 *Physical properties*

a. The vitreous weighs approximately 3.9 g
b. The volume of the vitreous is approximately 7 ml
c. The refractive index is 1.5
d. The vitreous is a hydro sol-gel structure
e. It does not transmit light below 300 nm

The vitreous is a hydro sol-gel structure weighing approximately 3.9 g and with a volume of 3.9 ml. The refractive index is similar to the aqueous (approximately 1.335). Most (90%) of visible light passes through the vitreous but transmission is zero in wavelengths less than 300 nm.

7.2 Structure

a. The vitreous framework is made of a specialised form of collagen
b. The collagen concentration is highest in the cortex
c. The hyaluronic acid concentration is responsible for the viscosity of the vitreous
d. The hyaluronic acid concentration is greatest in the cortex
e. Water content of the vitreous is 80% and is replaced every 10–15 hours

The framework of the vitreous is made up of a specialised type of collagen called vitrosin. This differs from normal collagen in that 49% of its weight is a complex polysaccharide and cannot be separated out. Hyaluronic acid, in the form of its sodium salt, accounts for the viscosity of the vitreous and (like vitrosin) is most concentrated in the cortex. Water makes up 98–99% of the vitreous and has a turnover time of 10–15 minutes.

7.3 Biochemistry

a. Sodium and potassium concentrations are approximately the same as those of the aqueous
b. The glucose concentration is highest at the retinal surface
c. The glycoprotein content is higher than the aqueous
d. Fluorescein is actively transported into the vitreous
e. Calcium soaps may be seen in the over 60s

Exchange of electrolytes occurs between the lens, retina, aqueous, and the vitreous but the electrolyte concentrations of the vitreous are approximately equal to those of the aqueous. Glucose concentrations are low at the retinal surface because it is used by the retina. The vitreous is rich in sialic acid. Its total glycoprotein content is five times greater than that of the aqueous. Fluorescein (and other anions) is actively transported out of the vitreous. Asteroid hyalosis is a condition seen after the sixth decade and is caused by calcium soaps in the vitreous.

7.4 *Properties of collagen*

a. Collagen is the most common protein in the animal world
b. Collagen is produced by fibroblasts
c. Type I collagen is found in the vitreous
d. Types I–III collagen are found in basement membranes
e. A collagen molecule is made of two separate polypeptide chains wrapped in a helix

Collagen, produced by fibroblasts, is the most common protein in the animal world and provides the extracellular framework for all multicellular organisms. A basic collagen unit (known as tropocollagen) is made of three polypeptide chains arranged in a left handed helix. Type I–III collagens are known as interstitial or fibrillar collagen; type I accounts for 80% of collagen in skin and 90% in bone; type II predominates in the vitreous. Types IV–XI do not form fibrils but appear as amorphous material in interstitial tissue or basement membranes.

7.5 *Collagen synthesis*

a. The initial stage is transcription and translation of the α chains
b. Each α chain has a triple repetitive amino acid sequence
c. Hydroxylation of proline occurs in the rough endoplasmic reticulum and is vitamin C dependent
d. The true fibrils are formed in the Golgi apparatus
e. Lysine oxidation results in cross linkages between α chains

Collagen synthesis is initiated by DNA transcription, followed by the processing of mRNA precursors and translation of the α chains (which have a triple repetitive amino acid sequence) in the ribosomes. The α chains move off the ribosomes into the cisternae of the rough endoplasmic reticulum, where modifications (such as the vitamin C dependent hydroxylation of proline and glycosylation) occur. The triple helix is formed in the rough endoplasmic reticulum and passes unchanged through the

Golgi apparatus. The terminal peptide chains are cleaved shortly after excretion from the cell. The critical extracellular modifications of collagen are lysine oxidation and formation of cross links—these are the main contributors to its tensile strength. Defects in lysine oxidation are seen in Marfan's syndrome.

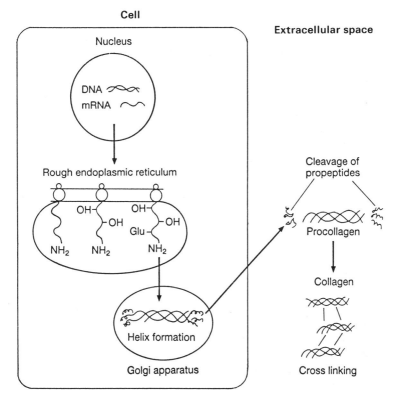

Fig 78 Steps in collagen synthesis

8: The pupil

8.1 *The normal pupil*

a. The diameter of the adult pupil can change from 2 to 9 mm
b. Simple anisocoria ($\leqslant 0.4$ mm) is found in 10% of the population
c. Simple anisocoria may change sides from day to day
d. The pupil is normally positioned slightly superonasally
e. Hippus refers to a physiological tremor

The pupil is capable of changing its diameter from 2 to 9 mm (an 87% change). Simple anisocoria is found in approximately 25% of the population and may change sides from day to day. The pupil is normally situated slightly inferonasally and has a physiological tremor, known as hippus.

8.2 *Pupillary reaction to light*

a. Latency, amplitude and duration of contraction all increase with increasing stimulus strength
b. Speed and size of contraction reach a plateau at 7–9 log units above the scotopic threshold
c. The latent period varies from 0.2 to 0.5 s (depending on the light source)
d. The pupil can respond to light frequencies up to 10 Hz
e. The pupillary reaction to light is quicker than that to accommodation

With light intensity up to 9 log units above threshold the strength and duration of pupillary contraction increases and latency period decreases. At intensities above 9 log units, the pupillary response plateaus off. The latent period is 0.2–0.5 s; less than that for constriction induced by accommodation. The pupil is not capable of responding to stimuli with a frequency greater than 5 Hz.

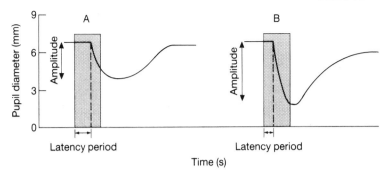

Fig 79 **Pupillary responses of dark adapted subjects. Intensity of flash A ≪ B**

8.3 *Effects of increasing pupil size*

a. A decreased depth of field
b. An increased depth of focus
c. An increased Stiles–Crawford effect
d. Decreased diffraction of light
e. Increased chromatic aberration

Pupillary dilation will decrease the depth of focus and depth of field, the converse being true for pupillary constriction. Light entering the eye at the edge of the pupil is less effective at stimulating photoreceptors than light entering at the centre. This is because of the shape of the receptors and the fact that light hits them obliquely, not axially. This effect (the Stiles–Crawford effect) is increased with mydriasis. As pupillary size increases diffraction of light decreases and chromatic aberration increases.

8.4 *Light reflexes*

a. The consensual reaction may be adequately tested even if that pupil is not visible
b. A unilateral optic nerve lesion will have a normal (consensual) indirect reflex
c. An impaired indirect pupillary reaction alone may be of no clinical significance
d. The light reflexes will be abnormal in occipital cortex lesions
e. Cataracts are a common cause of an afferent pupillary defect

The direct light reaction can not be tested adequately if the pupil being tested is not visible although the consensual reaction may be. An optic nerve lesion will not affect the efferent pupillary pathways, so the indirect light reflex will be normal. An impaired indirect pupillary reaction alone is usually of no clinical significance except as a potential source of confusion. Pupillary reflexes are brain stem reflexes and are therefore not affected by cortical lesions. Cataracts do not usually cause afferent pupillary defects; if cataract is present the prognosis for pseudophakic vision is generally poor.

8.5 *Efferent pupillary defects*

a. These defects characteristically present with a fixed constricted pupil
b. The lesion may also involve the red nucleus
c. Efferent pupillary defects will be found in lesions of the inferior colliculus
d. Defects may be caused by a posterior communicating artery aneurysm
e. Efferent pupillary defects are found in vascular third nerve lesions

Efferent pupillary defects characteristically present with a fixed dilated pupil. The causes of such a defect can broadly be grouped thus:
(1) Mid brain lesions, which may involve the red nucleus or the superior colliculus
(2) Third nerve lesions: if these are caused by compression from a posterior communicating artery aneurysm there will be pupillary involvement; those caused by vascular lesions are usually pupil sparing
(3) Lesions of the ciliary ganglion and short ciliary nerve
(4) Iris damage
(5) Drugs

8.6 *Efferent pupillary defects*

a. These defects may result from uncal herniation
b. Trauma to the ciliary ganglion may cause efferent pupillary defects
c. Efferent pupillary defects may be found with grossly raised intraocular pressure
d. Inadvertent exposure to a mydriatic may cause such defects
e. If an efferent pupillary defect is bilateral and associated with a vertical gaze palsy, it is caused by a dorsal mid brain lesion

Skull fractures to the pterion may damage the middle meningeal artery passing through a bony canal at this point, and cause an extradural haematoma. The resultant increase in intracranial pressure may produce mid brain displacement or transtentorial herniation of the uncus, resulting in a lesion to the third nerve. A large and sustained rise in intraocular pressure will cause hypoxia of the iris sphincter and will result in a fixed dilated pupil. A lesion of the dorsal mid brain will cause bilateral efferent pupillary defects with a vertical gaze palsy—this is known as Parinaud's syndrome or Sylvian aqueduct syndrome.

8.7 *Mydriasis*

a. Mydriasis is caused by cholinergic agonists
b. Mydriasis is caused by sympathomimetics
c. Phenylephrine produces mydriasis even in bright light
d. Phenylephrine produces a rebound miosis
e. Synthetic anticholinergics are more effective than belladonna alkaloids

Mydriasis is produced by contraction of the dilator pupillae, which is stimulated by noradrenergic sympathetic nerves that pass through the ciliary ganglion: sympathomimetic agents will therefore cause dilation. Cholinergic agents will constrict the pupil by stimulating the sphincter muscle. Phenylephrine (unlike atropine) is incapable of producing mydriasis in bright light and will produce a rebound miosis. Cocaine exerts its mydriatic effect by preventing noradrenaline reuptake. Synthetic anticholinergics such as homatropine and cyclopentolate are less effective mydriatics than belladonna alkaloids such as atropine.

8.8 *Mydriatic agents*

a. Heroin produces mydriasis
b. Nicotine produces mydriasis
c. Amphetamine produces mydriasis
d. Alcohol produces mydriasis
e. Cocaine causes mydriasis by increasing noradrenaline release from nerve terminals

Heroin will cause miosis (pinpoint pupils) by reducing the cortical inhibition of the Edinger–Westphal nucleus. Nicotine will produce mydriasis, as will alcohol. Amphetamine produces mydriasis by increasing noradrenaline release from nerve terminals: cocaine has a similar effect by preventing noradrenaline reuptake into the nerve terminals.

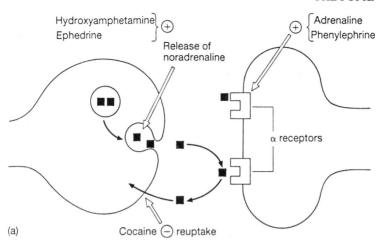

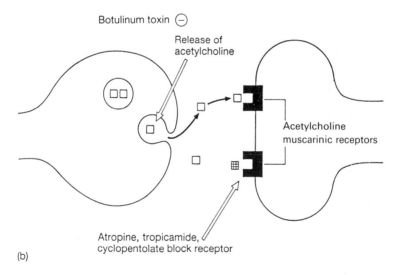

Fig 80 Mydriasis. (a) The adrenergic synapse and action of sympathomimetics; (b) the cholinergic synapse and actions of cholinergic blockade. ■, Noradrenaline; □, acetylcholine

233

8.9 *Causes of miosis*

Miosis is caused by:
a. Parasympathomimetics
b. Carbachol inhibiting acetylcholine release
c. Physostigmine
d. Thymoxamine
e. Hydroxyamphetamine

Stimulation of the sphincter pupillae via cholinergic postganglionic parasympathetic neurones from the ciliary ganglion causes miosis. Carbachol causes miosis by increasing acetylcholine release, whereas physostigmine has its effect by inhibiting acetylcholinesterases. Thymoxamine, an α adrenergic blocker, produces miosis by paralysing the dilator muscle. Hydroxyamphetamine increases noradrenaline release from nerve terminals and so causes mydriasis.

8.10 *Horner's syndrome*

a. Facial anhydrosis is not a feature of postganglionic Horner's syndrome
b. There is an increased anisocoria in dim light
c. Preganglionic lesions are usually more sinister than postganglionic lesions
d. Cocaine will dilate a Horner's pupil
e. Hydroxyamphetamine (1%) and adrenaline (1:1000) will both dramatically dilate the pupil in postganglionic lesions

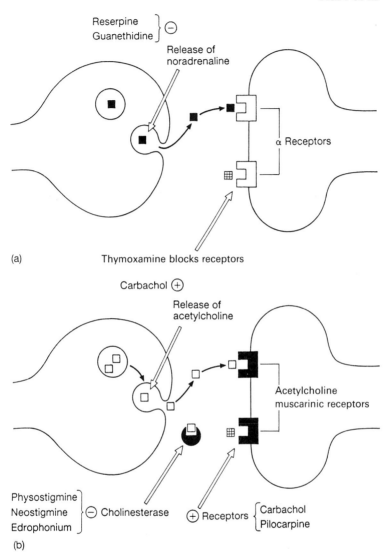

Fig 81 Miosis. (a) The adrenergic synapse and actions of sympathetic antagonists; (b) the cholinergic synapse and action of cholinomimetics

Horner's syndrome is caused by an interruption of the sympathetic chain in the head and neck and may be secondary to central (brain stem) lesions, preganglionic and postganglionic lesions. Anisocoria is increased in dim light because the normal pupil will dilate, whereas the Horner's pupil will not. The postganglionic sympathetic fibres that control facial sweating "travel" on the external (not the internal) carotid artery and are therefore not affected by a postganglionic Horner's syndrome. Preganglionic lesions are usually more sinister, being caused by lesions such as a Pancoast lung tumour. Pharmacological testing may be helpful, firstly in making the diagnosis of Horner's syndrome, and secondly in localising the lesion. Cocaine, which prevents the reuptake of noradrenaline at the adrenergic synapse, will not dilate a Horner's pupil but will cause dilatation in the normal eye. Hydroxyamphetamine will dilate a preganglionic or central Horner's pupil if the postganglionic pathway is intact. However, it will have no effect on a postganglionic Horner's pupil. There is no pharmacological test that can differentiate between a central and a preganglionic Horner's pupil. Postganglionic lesions exhibit denervation hypersensitivity and will therefore dilate with 1:1000 adrenaline.

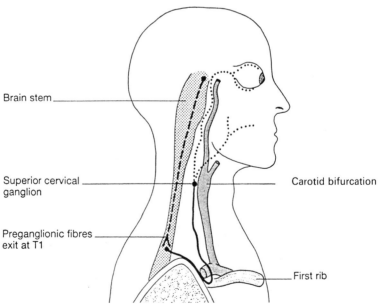

Brain stem

Superior cervical ganglion

Carotid bifurcation

Preganglionic fibres exit at T1

First rib

**Fig 82 Sympathetic supply to the eye. —— Preganglionic; – – – central; ....
postganglionic**

8.11 *Light near dissociation*

---

a. This is present only if the near response is greater than the response to bright light
b. Light near dissociation may be due to a normal light response and hyperactive near response
c. It is a feature of Horner's syndrome
d. Light near dissociation may be caused by a pretectal lesion
e. Light near dissociation may be seen in third nerve lesions

---

Light near dissociation is present only if the near response is greater than the response to bright light, and is always due to a diminished light response (not a hyperactive near response). Pretectal lesions, such as that seen in the Sylvian aqueduct syndrome, produce light near dissociation. Third nerve lesions can (surprisingly) cause a light near dissociation, not by sparing of "near" fibres but rather by aberrant reinnervation of the sphincter muscle by neurones normally supplying the medial rectus.

8.12 *Features of Argyll Robertson's pupils*

---

a. Argyll Robertson pupils are small
b. Argyll Robertson pupils may be confused with peripheral neuropathies
c. Physostigmine causes increased constriction
d. Atropine causes dilation
e. The lesion is situated in the ciliary ganglion

The Argyll Robertson pupil was originally described in 1869 in a series of patients with tabes dorsalis. These patients had light sensitive retinas, a good pupillary near response but did not respond to light. The pupils were small, did not dilate with atropine and constricted further with physostigmine. The exact site of the lesion is not known but is thought to be in the vicinity of the pretectal nuclei.

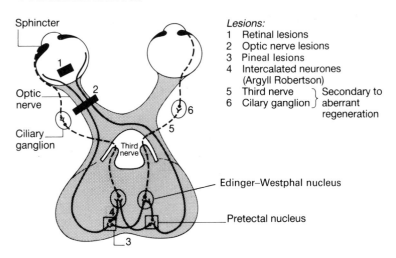

Sphincter

Optic nerve

Ciliary ganglion

Third nerve

Lesions:
1 Retinal lesions
2 Optic nerve lesions
3 Pineal lesions
4 Intercalated neurones (Argyll Robertson)
5 Third nerve ⎫ Secondary to
6 Cilary ganglion ⎭ aberrant regeneration

Edinger–Westphal nucleus

Pretectal nucleus

Fig 83 Sympathetic supply to the eye. – – – Preganglionic; —— central

8.13 *Features of Adie's pupils*

a. Adie's pupils exhibit light near dissociation
b. Adie's pupils are supersensitive to cholinergics
c. Blurred vision is often a presenting symptom
d. Involvement of the second eye is often unnoticed by the patient
e. The lesion is thought to involve the Edinger-Westphal nucleus

The light reaction of Adie's pupils is sluggish and the near response is usually strong and tonic. The supersensitivity to cholinergics is a post denervation phenomenon, as this condition is produced by a ciliary ganglion lesion. The first symptom is usually blurred vision caused by accommodative paresis. If the second eye becomes involved the patient (often in her late 40s) might not notice this loss of accommodation.

9: The extraocular muscles and ocular movements

9.1 *Frames of reference and gaze positions*

a. The fixed point of the centre of rotation is 13.5 mm posterior to the corneal apex
b. The fixed point of the centre of rotation is 1.6 mm to the temporal side of the geometric centre
c. Movement to the secondary position involves rotation about X or Z axes
d. The tertiary position is achieved by movement around the X and Z axes simultaneously
e. Tertiary gaze positions are associated with true torsion

The fixed point of the centre of rotation is 13.5 mm posterior to the corneal apex and 1.6 mm to the nasal side of the geometric centre. Fick's axes include a horizontal X axis, a horizontal Y axis (90° to the X, which passes through the pupil) and a vertical Z axis. The secondary gaze positions are achieved by rotation around the X or Z axes, whereas tertiary gaze or oblique positions are achieved by simultaneous rotation about the X and Z axes. The torsional movements associated with tertiary gaze positions are false.

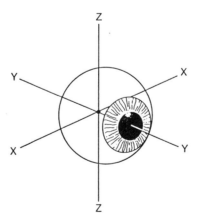

Fig 84 Fick's axes

239

9.2 *Muscle action in the isolated agonist model*

a. The primary action of medial rectus is adduction
b. The primary action of superior oblique is depression
c. The primary action of superior rectus is elevation
d. The primary action of inferior oblique is excyclotorsion
e. The primary action of inferior rectus is depression

The primary action of the muscle in the isolated agonist model is that movement which occurs when the muscle contracts with the eye in the primary position. The medial rectus is an adductor and has no secondary actions. The superior oblique is primarily an incyclotortor, but when adducted to 54° its prime action is depression. The inferior oblique's primary action is excyclotorsion and it is an elevator in adduction. The superior and inferior recti muscles are primarily elevators and depressors respectively.

9.3 *The following are yoked muscles*

a. Right lateral rectus, left medial rectus
b. Right superior rectus, left inferior oblique
c. Right superior oblique, left inferior oblique
d. Right inferior rectus, left superior oblique
e. Right inferior oblique, left superior rectus

Yoked muscles contract to move both eyes in the same direction, that is, the right lateral rectus and left medial rectus both move the eyes to the right. The superior oblique on the right and inferior rectus on the left moves the eyes down and to the left. The right inferior rectus and the left superior oblique move the eyes down and to the right.

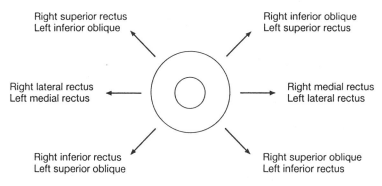

Fig 85 Extraocular muscles: the cardinal positions of gaze

9.4 *Torsional movements*

a. The torsional effect of the superior rectus is maximal with lateral gaze
b. The torsional effect of the inferior rectus increases with medial gaze
c. The superior rectus causes incyclotorsion
d. The inferior rectus causes incyclotorsion
e. The amount of false torsion associated with any tertiary position of gaze is constant regardless of how the eye achieved that position

The superior rectus causes elevation (which is maximal if the eye is abducted 24°), and incyclotorsion (which is maximal on adduction or medial gaze). The inferior rectus causes depression (which is maximal in 24° of abduction) and excyclotorsion (which is maximal in adduction). Donder's law states that the amount of false torsion associated with any tertiary position of gaze is constant, regardless of how the eye achieved that position.

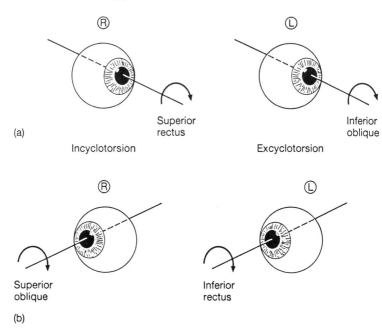

Fig 86 Torsional movements: (a) left gaze; (b) right gaze

9.5 *Control of extraocular movement*

a. The semicircular canals detect rotational movements
b. The semicircular canals connect with the inferior and medial vestibular nuclei
c. The utricle and the saccule detect head tilting movements
d. The floculonodular lobe is intimately involved with the vestibular input to the extraocular muscles
e. The vestibulospinal inputs are of prime importance in the regulation of the extraocular muscle position

The semicircular canals detect rotatory movements of the head and connect with the superior and medial vestibular nuclei. The utricle and saccule detect head tilting (gravitational effects) and connect with the inferior and medial nuclei. The floculonodular lobe of the cerebellum mediates vestibular inputs to the oculomotor system, whereas the vermis is involved with initiation of eye movements. Although vestibular spinal inputs from cervical proprioceptors play an important role in controlling eye movements in certain mammals, they are of minimal importance in humans.

9.6 *Influences on extraocular muscle control*

> a. The superior colliculus is retinotopically mapped
> b. The superior colliculus responds to auditory stimulation
> c. The vermis is involved with initiation of eye movements
> d. Frontal eye fields mediate contralateral saccadic eye movements
> e. The inferior colliculus is connected to the extraocular muscle nuclei

The superior colliculus is retinotopically mapped and is connected to the extraocular muscle nuclei, unlike the inferior colliculus which is involved in auditory pathways. The cerebellar vermis is involved with initiation of eye movements, and the frontal eye fields mediate contralateral saccadic eye movements.

9.7 *Version and vergence*

> a. Hering's law applies to vergence movements
> b. Version movements are quicker than vergence movements
> c. Retinal disparity is a stimulus for version movements
> d. Section of the corpus callosum inhibits vergence
> e. Version movements form part of the near triad

In versional movements the eyes move in the same direction—
the visual axes of the eyes remain parallel. Hering's law states
that in all voluntary conjugate movements equal and simultaneous innervation flows from ocular motor centres to the muscles
establishing the direction of gaze. Vergence movements are
slower than versional movements, are stimulated by retinal
disparity (as opposed to blur), and are inhibited by section of
the corpus callosum. They also form part of the near triad.

9.8 Smooth pursuit movements

a. The function of smooth pursuit movement is to keep an
   object of interest on the fovea
b. The maximum velocity of these movements is 20° per
   second
c. Occipital lobe lesions lead to loss of smooth pursuit to the
   ipsilateral side
d. Frontal lobe lesions lead to loss of smooth pursuit to the
   contralateral side
e. Smooth pursuit movements have a latency of 50 ms

Smooth pursuit movements are designed to keep an object of
interest on the fovea. They have a velocity of up to 100° per
second, a latency of 125 ms and (along with saccadic movements) are seen in opticokinetic nystagmus. They are controlled
by the occipital cortex, destruction of which will cause loss of
smooth pursuit to the ipsilateral side. Frontal lobe lesions have
no effect on smooth pursuit movements.

9.9 Saccadic movements

a. The usual stimulus is an object of interest in the peripheral visual field
b. Saccadic movements have a maximum velocity of 400° per
   second
c. Saccadic movements are produced by "burst-tonic"
   neurones
d. Saccadic movements are initiated by the frontal cortex
e. Visual threshold increases during saccades

Saccadic movements are designed to place an object of interest in the peripheral visual field on to the fovea. They are the fastest of all eye movements, with a velocity of up to 400° per second and are controlled by the frontal cortex. The neurones involved are "burst-tonic" neurones, which produce a biphasic movement. The initial "pulse" phase and the following "step" phase are matched by the floculus to produce a smooth movement. During the saccade there is an increase in the visual threshold.

9.10 *Fixation movements*

a. Drifts are binocular
b. Microsaccades are monocular
c. Tremors may have a frequency of up to 80 Hz
d. Drifts have a maximum amplitude of 30'
e. The amplitude of tremors is approximately 10–30' of arc

Fixation movements are designed to move the retinal image by very small distances at regular intervals and prevent the image fading due to persistent bleaching of photoreceptor pigments (Troxler's phenomenon). Drifts are monocular and have a maximum amplitude of 6'. Microsaccades are binocular. Tremors can have a frequency of up to 80 Hz and have an amplitude of 10–30" of arc.

9.11 *Optokinetic nystagmus*

a. Optokinetic nystagmus is a mixture of saccadic and slow movements
b. Optokinetic nystagmus may be elicited by a striped drum revolving at speeds of 30–200° per second
c. Optokinetic nystagmus is an accurate test of visual acuity
d. Direction of initial eye movement varies according to the attentiveness of the subject
e. A central scotoma decreases the maximum speed at which optokinetic nystagmus may be elicited

Optokinetic nystagmus is a biphasic movement that can be elicited by a striped drum revolving at 30–100° per second. The smooth pursuit component is a compensatory movement and is followed by a quicker saccadic movement. To elicit optokinetic nystagmus the patient must be attentive: if he or she pays particular attention to the drum, the initial movement is saccadic (predictive in the direction to which the stripe entered the peripheral field); if not, the initial movement is compensatory in the direction of the revolving drum. Optokinetic drums may be used as a crude measure of visual acuity, and may be useful in cases of "hysterical" visual loss. The presence of a central scotoma will increase the frequency at which optokinetic nystagmus can be elicited.

9.12 *Vestibulo-ocular reflexes and caloric testing*

a. Stimulation of a semicircular canal leads to nystagmus in the plane of that canal
b. The slow phase is always in the same direction as the movement causing the nystagmus
c. Hot water in the right ear causes nystagmus with a quick phase to the right
d. Cold water in the left ear causes nystagmus with a slow phase to the left
e. Bilateral stimulation causes vertical nystagmus

Floren's law states that stimulation of a semicircular canal leads to nystagmus in the plane of that canal, the slow phase of which is always in a direction opposite to that causing the nystagmus. The direction of the nystagmus always refers to the fast saccadic component. With a patient's head held backwards at 60° the horizontal canal predominates and caloric testing may be carried out. Warm water causes the endolymph to rise in the horizontal canal, stimulating the end organ. This is equivalent to an ipsilateral head turn and causes a smooth eye movement to the contralateral side, which is followed by a corrective fast saccadic movement to the ipsilateral side. The opposite is true if cold water is used (cold opposite warm same: COWS) Vertical nystagmus will be elicited by bilateral stimulation.

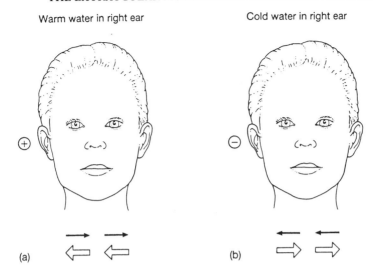

Fig 87 Caloric testing: (a) stimulation of the right horizontal canal; (b) inhibition of the right horizontal canal. → Slow phase; ⇨ fast saccadic movement

9.13 *The following reduce the response to caloric testing*

a. Fixation on an object
b. Darkness
c. Opticokinetic stimuli
d. High plus lenses
e. Decreased visual acuity

The response to caloric testing is reduced by fixating strongly on an object and by an opticokinetic stimulus. Darkness and high plus lenses will stimulate the response but decreased visual acuity has no effect.

10: The retina

10.1 Retinal metabolism

a. The respiratory rate of the retina is twice that of the brain
b. Glucose stores are adequate for 1 hour
c. Lactate will accumulate even if adequate oxygen is present
d. Müller cells have glucose 6 phosphatase activity
e. Myoid regions of the photoreceptors are rich in mitochondria

The respiratory rate of the retina is twice that of the brain. Half of the respiratory rate is accounted for by the ellipsoid regions of the photoreceptors, which are rich in mitochondria. Unlike the brain, the retina does not require insulin for glucose to enter into the cells. Müller cells possess glucose 6 phosphatase activity, which enables them to release glucose from their "stores" into the neuroretina. Glycolysis occurs even if there is a sufficient supply of oxygen (unlike other tissues): this causes an accumulation of lactate.

10.2 Glycolysis

a. Glycolysis produces a net gain of two ATPs
b. Phosphofructokinase is the rate determining enzyme in glycolysis
c. Glycolysis in the retina does not occur in the presence of oxygen
d. Glycolysis occurs in mitochondria
e. Glucose 6 phosphatase and hexokinase catalyse the same reaction in opposite directions

Glycolysis is the process by which glucose is converted to pyruvate and lactate. It produces a net gain of two ATPs and in most tissues occurs only if there is no oxygen present, the retina being an exception to this "rule". Phosphofructokinase catalyses the conversion of fructose 6 phosphate to fructose 1, 6 biphosphate, which is the rate determining step in glycolysis. This reaction is indirectly influenced by hormones such as glucagon. Hexokinase catalyses the conversion of glucose to glucose 6 phospate; the opposite reaction is catalysed by glucose 6 phosphatase. All these reactions occur in the cytoplasm.

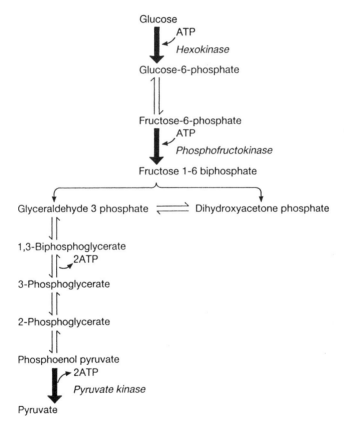

Fig 88 Glycolysis. ⬇ Rate determining steps

10.3 *The Krebs' citric acid cycle*

a. This cycle requires oxygen
b. The Krebs' cycle produces an ATP yield that is 18 times greater than that of glycolysis
c. This cycle involves the coupling of oxaloacetate and acetyl coenzyme A to produce citrate
d. For every two hydrogen ions liberated three ATP are produced via oxidative phosphorylation
e. Oxidative phosphorylation occurs in the outer mitochondrial membrane

The Krebs' citric acid cycle is the process by which citric acid (a six carbon sugar formed by the coupling of oxaloacetate and acetyl coenzyme A) is converted to a four carbon sugar, releasing hydrogen ions and ATP. This occurs on the inner mitochondrial membrane. For every two hydrogen ions released three ATPs are produced by oxidative phosphorylation. The cycle requires oxygen, and for every glucose molecule fed into the system in glyclolysis there is a net production of 36 ATPs.

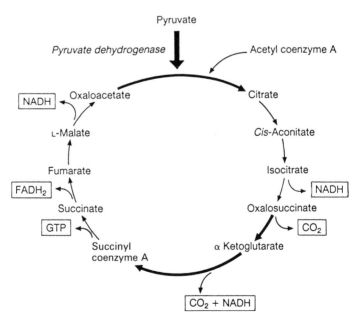

Fig 89 Krebs' citric acid cycle. ➡ **Rate determining step**

10.4 *Gluconeogenesis*

a. Gluconeogenesis is glycolysis in reverse
b. Gluconeogenesis is strongly influenced by glucagon
c. Transamination is the first step in the conversion of amino acids to glucose
d. Glycerol is converted to glucose via dihydroxyacetone phosphate
e. Gluconeogenesis occurs predominantly in the liver

Gluconeogenesis is the production of glucose from non-carbohydrate sources. It is not just the reverse of glycolysis, as several reactions are catalysed by enzymes different from those involved in glycolysis. These gluconeogenic enzymes are influenced by the action of glucagon. Proteins can be converted to glucose, the first step being transamination of amino acids; glycerol may also be converted to glucose via dihydroxyacetone phosphate. Gluconeogenesis occurs predominantly in the liver.

10.5 *The pentose phosphate pathway*

a. This pathway is essential for RNA and DNA production
b. The pentose phosphate pathway is reversibly linked with the glycolytic pathway
c. NADPH is generated by the pentose phosphate pathway
d. The pentose phosphate pathway does not occur in the retina
e. The pentose phosphate pathway encompasses the Cori cycle

The pentose phosphate pathway is the alternative route for metabolism of glucose and is important in the production of intermediates for RNA and DNA. It is reversibly linked at a number of stages to the glycolytic pathway and is important in generating NADPH. The pentose phosphate pathway is an integral part of retinal metabolism, in combination with glycolysis and the Krebs' citric acid cycle. The Cori cycle is involved in recycling lactate to glucose by the liver and is independent of the pentose phosphate shunt.

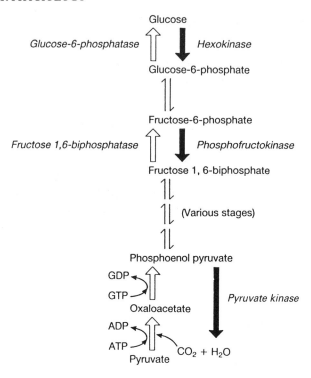

Fig 90 Gluconeogenesis (⇨) versus glycolysis (➡)

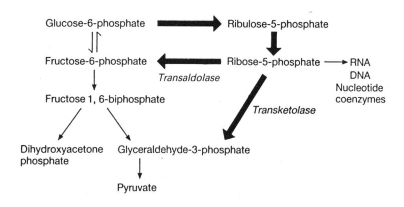

Fig 91 The pentose phosphate pathway (➡)

10.6 *Properties of vitamin A*

a. Vitamin A is a fat soluble vitamin
b. Adult daily requirement of vitamin A is 2500 IU
c. Deficiency of vitamin A can cause growth retardation
d. Vitamin A deficiency can cause corneal vascularisation
e. 1% of the body's vitamin A is stored in the retina

Vitamin A is a fat soluble vitamin (as are vitamins D, E, and K), the daily adult requirement of which is 2500 IU. Deficiency may cause growth retardation, xerophthalmia, corneal vascularisation and night blindness. Only 0.01% of the body's total vitamin A is stored in the retina, the main store being the liver.

10.7 *Metabolism of vitamin A*

a. Retinal pigment epithelial cells have receptors for retinol binding protein
b. Conversion of 11-*cis*-retinal to all-*trans*-retinal involves a conformational change
c. The recombination of 11-*cis* isomers and opsin is enzymatic
d. Esterification of retinal occurs in the neural layer of the retina
e. Small amounts of retinal are lost by peroxidase degradation

Retinol is found in the plasma bound to a specific binding protein, for which the retinal pigment epithelial cells have receptors. Its aldehyde form, retinal, passes from the retinal pigment epithelium to the photoreceptors, where its derivative, 11-*cis*-retinal forms the chromophore portion of all four visual pigments. The electrophysiological response of the photoreceptor to light is triggered by photons, which by a process of photoisomerisation convert 11-*cis*-retinal to all-*trans*-retinal. The all-*trans*-retinal dislodges from the surface of the opsin molecule. It is unclear whether the conversion of all-*trans*-retinal back to the 11-*cis* isomer is enzymic, but the latter spontaneously recombines with opsin. Following photolysis the all-*trans*-retinal is reduced to all-*trans*-retinol by a retinol dehydrogenase in the photoreceptor outer segments. Much of the retinol now diffuses into the retinal pigment epithelium, transport that may be aided by interstitial retinol binding protein. If left to accumulate retinol would adversely affect membrane stability, so it is esterified to render it safe for intracellular storage. Most of the retinoid is recycled in the above manner, but a small fraction is lost through diffusion or by peroxidase degradation.

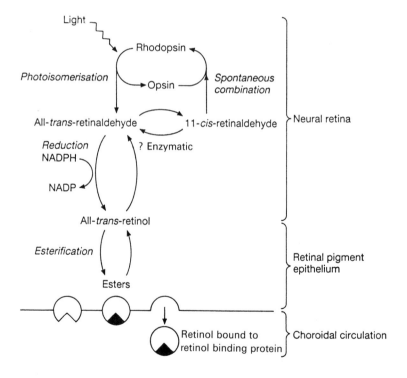

Fig 92 Vitamin A metabolism in the retina

10.8 *Photochemistry of the mammalian retina*

> a. The conversion of rhodopsin to bathorhodopsin is the only photoreaction in the retina
> b. The conversion of metarhodopsin I to metarhodopsin II is reversible
> c. Sodium continues to be extruded from the inner segments of photoreceptors irrespective of light conditions
> d. The concentration of cyclic GMP is highest in the dark
> e. Adenylate cyclase activity influences cyclic GMP concentrations

The conversion of rhodopsin to bathorhodopsin is the only photoreaction in the retina, the others being thermal reactions. The only reversible reaction is that between metarhodopsin I and II. Metarhodopsin catalyses the conversion of T.GDP to T.GTP, which in turn activates phosphodiesterase. Cyclic GMP controls the entrance of sodium into the photoreceptor outer segments, although sodium is continuously extruded from the inner segments. Cyclic GMP levels are governed by the activity of adenylate cyclase, and are highest in scotopic conditions when the photoreceptors are depolarised. In photopic conditions adenylate cyclase (stimulated by phosphodiesterase) converts cyclic GMP to 5'GMP. This results in closure of outer segment sodium channels and photoreceptor hyperpolarisation.

10.9 *Retinal circulation*

> a. Photoreceptors receive nutrients from the choroidal vessels
> b. The retinal vessels supply nutrients to the inner plexiform layer
> c. Retinal vessels have a sympathetic innervation
> d. Venous pulsation is secondary to changes in intraocular pressure
> e. Choroidal blood flow per 100 g is ten times greater than that of grey matter

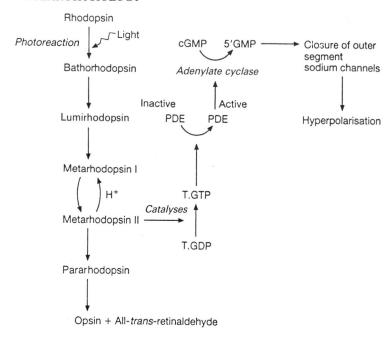

Fig 93 Phototransduction. T, Transduction; PDE, phosphodiesterase

The inner two thirds of the retina, down to and including the inner portion of the inner nuclear layer, receives nutrients from the retinal vessels. The outer third, which includes the photoreceptors, receives nutrients from the choroidal circulation. The central retinal artery does not have any sympathetic innervation beyond the lamina cribrosa; blood flow is therefore controlled by autoregulation. The pressure in the retinal veins is approximately equal to that of the intraocular pressure. During systole the intraocular pressure is increased by the increasing blood volume, which causes the apparent venous pulsation. The choroidal blood flow is ten times greater than that of grey matter.

10.10 *Metabolism of melanin*

a. The conversion of tyrosine to dopa is the rate determining step
b. Conversion of dopa to dopaquinone is non-enzymatic
c. Polymerisation of 5-6 dihydroxyindole produces melanin
d. Melanin is not found in tissues derived from the neuroretina
e. Melanin has stable free radicals which can accept electrons

The production of melanin is an "offshoot" of tyrosine metabolism, the rate determining step being the conversion of tyrosine to dopa by tyrosine hydroxylase. The conversion of dopa to dopaquinone is non-enzymatic. The final step in the pathway involves the polymerisation of 5–6 dihydroxyindole to produce melanin. Melanin is found in the posterior pigmented iris epithelium, which is derived from the neuroretina. Melanin has stable free radicals that undergo dipolar reactions with water to produce characteristic magnetic resonance images.

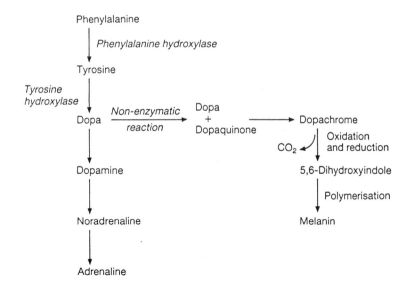

Fig 94 Melanin metabolism

10.11 *Functions of the retinal pigment epithelium*

a. The retinal pigment epithelium acts as a solar screen
b. Retinol and its derivatives are stored in the retinal pigment epithelium
c. The retinal pigment epithelium phagocytoses photoreceptor outer segments forms part of the blood retinal barrier
d. The retinal pigment epithelium forms part of the blood retinal barrier
e. The retinal pigment epithelium is responsible for b wave of the electroretinogram

The retinal pigment epithelium is composed of cells rich in melanosomes and lysosomes with microvilli that project between the photoreceptor cells. Because of its melanin content it functions as a solar screen and it is involved in photoreceptor outer segment phagocytosis. The tight junctions between epithelial cells are an integral part of the blood brain barrier. Ionic imbalance across its cells produces the c wave of the electroretinogram.

10.12 *Properties and functions of Müller cells*

a. Müller cells have a supportive function
b. Müller cells form part of the external limiting membrane
c. Glucose and retinoids are stored in Müller cells
d. These cells may have phagocytic functions
e. Müller cells are responsible for the c wave of the electroretinogram

The Müller cells are glial cells and as such their primary role is supportive. The expanded terminations and basement membrane of these cells form the internal limiting membrane. Junctions between the photoreceptor cells and the radial processes of the Müller cells forms the external limiting membrane. They are capable of storing glucose and retinoids, and in some pathological states may assume a phagocytic role. Müller cells are also responsible for the b wave of the electroretinogram.

10.13 *Properties of photoreceptors*

a. Photoreceptors are derived from ciliated ependymal cells
b. The myoid region is predominantly involved in synthesis
c. All cones are conical in shape
d. Most cone disc laminae are continuous with the extracellular space
e. There are approximately 1000 rod outer segment lamellae

Photoreceptors are derived from clinical ependymal cells of the neuroectoderm. The myoid region is involved in synthesis, the elipsoid region with energy production. Characteristically cones were described as being conical in shape but this is not true of all cones. Most cone lamellae (unlike rod outer segment lamellae) are in continuity with the extracellular space. Approximately 1000 lamellae are present at any one time in the rod outer segment.

10.14 *Turnover of photoreceptors*

a. Photoreceptor turnover can be studied with radiolabelled amino acids
b. Shedding of rod discs peaks at dusk
c. Outer segment turnover time is 9–13 days
d. Shedding of cone discs peaks first thing in the morning
e. Rod and cone shedding is influenced by hormones

Photoreceptor segments are in a continuous state of flux. Young and coworkers in 1976 studied photoreceptor cell renewal with radiolabelled amino acids and showed that rod outer segment turnover time is approximately 9–13 days. Rod disc shedding is at a maximum in the morning and cone shedding is maximal at dusk. Both are influenced by melatonin whose production has a diurnal pattern.

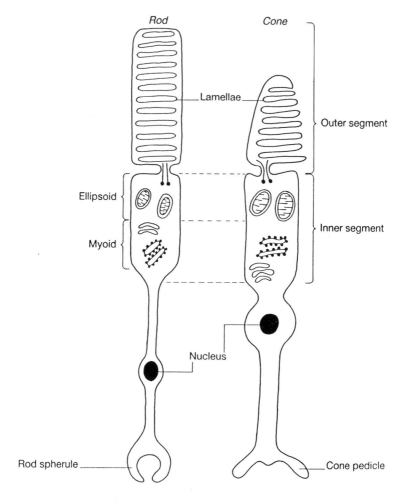

Fig 95 Structure of rods and cones

10.15 *Neurotransmitters*

> a. Acetylcholine is found in relatively low concentrations in the inner plexiform layer
> b. Concentrations of γ-aminobutyric acid are increased by light
> c. L-aspartate may be the transmitter for rods and cones
> d. Noradrenaline is found in amacrine cells
> e. Glycine is an inhibitory peptide found in the retina

Acetylcholine is probably the transmitter at the bipolar synapse and is found in high concentrations in the inner plexiform layer. Although the exact role of γ-aminobutyric acid is not known its levels increase in photopic conditions. Glycine is an inhibitory peptide found in the amacrine cells. Noradrenaline is not found in the retina. The retinal transmitter between photoreceptors and bipolar cells has not been elucidated, but L-aspartate is the favoured choice at present.

11: Electrodiagnostic tests

11.1 *The electroretinogram*

> a. The electroretinogram is an electrical mass response of the retina
> b. The a wave is produced by the photoreceptor cells
> c. The b wave is produced by the retinal pigment epithelial cells
> d. The b wave implicit time is the time between onset of the stimulus and peak of the b wave
> e. The b wave implicit time is the difference between the peak of the a wave and peak of the b wave

The electroretinogram was first described in the 19th century by Holmgren. A clinical recording technique was developed by Riggs (1941) and Karpe (1945) using corneal electrodes mounted in haptic contact lenses. Its major components in response to a single bright white flash are the a and b waves, which vary in amplitude and timing according to the adaptive state of the eye and the type of stimulus. The a wave is a cornea negative deflection that is thought to be generated in the photoreceptor cells. This is followed by the larger cornea positive b wave which is generated in the Müller cells, which act as a "sink" for potassium ions released by depolarising bipolar cells. For most clinical purposes these are the main components that are considered. Superimposed upon the b wave is a series of fast wavelets known as the oscillatory potentials which have limited clinical value. The slower c wave (a positive component generated in the pigment epithelium), and the d wave (an off-response following the cessation of constant illumination) are rarely used in routine clinical practice. The ganglion cells make no contribution to the flash electroretinogram. Measurement comprises the implicit time or latency of the components, from the onset of the stimulus to the peak (or trough) of the component concerned, and the amplitude of the a and b waves. The a wave amplitude is measured from onset, the b wave amplitude from the peak (or trough—the electroretinogram is usually displayed with positivity upwards) of the a wave.

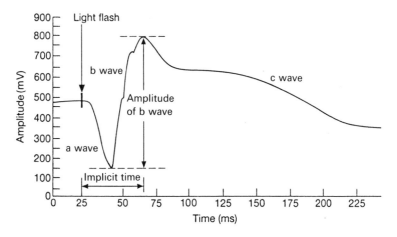

Fig 96 Dark adapted response to a flash electroretinogram

11.2 *Photopic, scotopic and flicker electroretinograms*

a. With a bright white flash stimulus the amplitude of the a
   wave is maximal in scotopic conditions
b. With a bright white flash stimulus the amplitude of the b
   wave is maximal in photopic conditions
c. A very dim blue or white stimulus in scotopic conditions
   will give a pure rod electroretinogram
d. Cone dystrophies have an abnormal flicker electroretinogram
e. Retinitis pigmentosa will give a normal scotopic electroretinogram

With the standard bright white flash a mixed rod–cone electroretinogram is recorded, both a and b wave amplitudes being
maximal in the dark adapted eye. When a very dim white or blue
flash is used in scotopic conditions the response is generated
purely by the rods. In contrast, a cone response can be recorded
with a bright white light superimposed upon a rod-saturating
background, or with a 30 Hz flicker stimulus. The rods have
poor temporal resolution and are unable to respond to a stimulus presented at this rate. Retinitis pigmentosa is primarily a
disease of the rods, and will affect the scotopic electroretinogram. Congenital night blindness produces a characteristic
"negative" electroretinograph, which is caused by abolition of
the rod b wave, probably due to a selective block at the rod
bipolar synapse. This abnormality is also seen in retinoschisis,
and is a classic sign. The rods apparently function normally. In
early cone abnormalities the increase of the implicit time is often
unaccompanied by any reduction in amplitude.

263

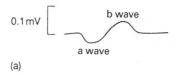

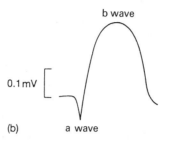

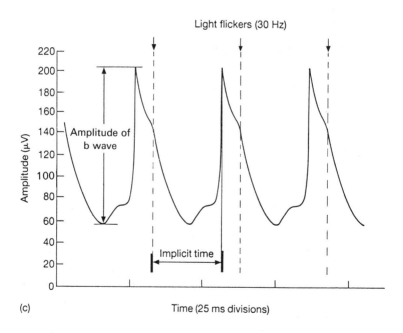

Fig 97 Photopic a and b waves (a), scotopic a and b waves (b), and flicker electroretinogram (c)

11.3 *Pattern electroretinograms*

Pattern electroretinograms are :
a. Produced by bipolar cells
b. Produced by ganglion cells
c. Produced by optic nerve activity
d. Generated by the macula
e. In glaucoma the pattern electroretinogram is normal

The pattern electroretinogram consists of two main components, P_{50} and N_{95}. The letter refers to the positive or negative polarity of the response, and the subscript to the timing (ms) of the peak of the response. P_{50} is produced by damage to the inner retina and ganglion cells and N_{95} is selectively affected by optic nerve damage. The amplitude/unit area of the pattern electroretinogram varies with the cell density and therefore less dominated by the fovea than the visual evoked potential. It is abnormal in a variety of local macular conditions and early retinal degenerations.

11.4 *Uses of the electroretinogram*

a. Distinction between localised and diffuse retinal disease
b. Distinction between retinal and optic nerve disease
c. Distinction between macular and optic nerve disease
d. Distinction between disease affecting the choroidal circulation and the central retinal artery circulation
e. Estimation of visual acuity

As the flash electroretinogram is an electrical mass response of the retina, it is unaffected by a small localised lesion and will be normal in disease confined to the macula. The ganglion cells make no contribution to the (flash) electroretinogram, which may be used to distinguish between generalised retinal disease and optic nerve disease but not between macular and optic neuropathy. The photoreceptors are supplied via the choroidal circulation whereas the bipolar cells are supplied via the central retinal artery: both a and b waves are affected in choroidal disease but the a wave is spared in, for example, central retinal artery occlusion. The electroretinogram cannot be used to determine visual acuity.

265

11.5 *The electro-oculogram*

a. The electro-oculogram uses fixed excursion lateral eye movements to measure the corneoretinal standing potential

b. The electro-oculogram is measured with a skin and scleral contact lens electrode

c. The electro-oculogram is measured in light adaptation followed by dark adaptation

d. The electro-oculogram reflects retinal pigment epithelial activity

e. The critical value is the absolute peak voltage seen following light adaptation

The electro-oculogram measures the corneoretinal standing potential by using fixed excursion lateral eye movements in conditions of varying luminance. Measurements between pairs of electrodes at the outer and inner canthi are taken during dark adaptation (approximately 20 min) followed by adaptation to a bright light for a slightly shorter period. The amplitude of the signal reaches a minimum in dark (the dark trough) and should increase markedly during light adaptation to a maximum value (the light peak). The critical value is the ratio between the light peak and dark trough (the Arden ratio), normally expressed as a percentage, and is usually greater than 180% in normal eyes.

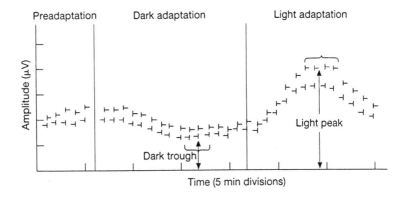

Fig 98 The electro-oculogram. ⊢ **Right eye;** ⊣ **left eye**

11.6 Uses of the electro-oculogram

The electro-oculogram:
a. Can distinguish between localised and diffuse retinal disease
b. Establishes retinal integrity in the presence of opaque media
c. Can distinguish between rod and cone dysfunction
d. Can distinguish between macular and optic nerve disease
e. Always parallels the electroretinogram

In general the results of the electro-oculogram will parallel those of the electroretinogram, a notable exception being the case of vitelliform macular dystrophy, where the electroretinogram is normal and the electro-oculogram light rise is remarkably reduced. It is, therefore, useful in distinguishing between localised and diffuse retinal disease and for establishing retinal integrity in the presence of opaque media. However, as it is a function of retinal pigment epithelial activity, the electro-oculogram cannot distinguish between rod and cone dysfunction or between macular and optic nerve disease.

11.7 The pattern electroretinogram

a. The pattern electroretinogram is generated in the outer retinal layers
b. The pattern electroretinogram reflects retinal ganglion cell activity
c. The pattern electroretinogram can distinguish between macular and optic nerve disease
d. The pattern electroretinogram will always be abnormal in optic nerve disease
e. The pattern electroretinogram is useful in the management of ocular hypertension

The first report that small retinal potentials are evoked when a pattern is reversed in contrast was made by Riggs in 1964. The main components of the transient pattern electroretinogram in response to a reversing checkerboard stimulus (2–6 reversals per second) are a positive component (P_{50}), at approximately 50 ms, and a larger negative component (N_{95}) at approximately 95 ms. The disappearance in the cat of the pattern electroretinogram following optic nerve section, in association with the development of retinal ganglion cell degeneration, implicated the ganglion cells in the origins of the pattern electroretinogram, but recent work in humans shows that the P_{50} and N_{95} components are different. It seems likely that N_{95} and some of P_{50} are ganglion cell derived, but that there may be a significant contribution to the P_{50} component from more distal retina. The pattern electroretinogram is derived from central retina and the P_{50} component is almost invariably abnormal in macular dysfunction. In contrast, optic nerve disease will affect the pattern electroretinogram only if there has been significant retrograde degeneration to the retinal ganglion cells—and then the abnormality may occur only in the N_{95} component. An abnormal pattern electroretinogram in a patient with ocular hypertension suggests that the patient may be developing glaucoma.

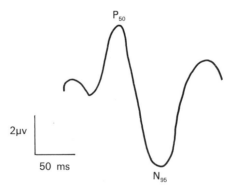

Fig 99 The pattern electroretinogram

11.8 *Visual evoked potentials*

a. The visual evoked potential is a measure of the occipital cortices electrical response to visual stimulation
b. Pupillary dilation must be performed to measure the visual evoked potential
c. The stimulus is usually a bright white flash
d. When recording the visual evoked potential, refractive error must always be corrected
e. The visual evoked potential can be used to assess the function of the optic nerves and optic chiasm

The visual evoked potential is a measure of the response of the occipital cortex to visual stimulation. It is extracted, using scalp electrodes, from the background electroencephalographic activity by the computerised averaging of the responses to repeated stimuli. The usual stimuli are a reversing checkerboard pattern or, perhaps less routinely, a diffuse flash. Pupillary dilation is contraindicated for pattern visual evoked potentials, due to the resulting loss of accommodation. Correction of refractive error is necessary for recording the pattern visual evoked potential, but the flash visual evoked potential is unaffected by defocussing, and does not require the cooperation of the patient to the extent demanded for successful pattern visual evoked potential recording. The flash visual evoked potential can be used in uncooperative patients such as infants or preverbal infants or patients who are unconscious or in coma. Provided that multiple recording channels are used in conjunction with appropriate stimuli (often hemifield pattern stimuli) assessment of both optic nerve and chiasmal function is possible.

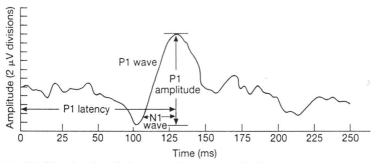

Fig 100 **The visual evoked potential in a normal subject**

269

11.9 *The visual evoked potential waveform*

a. The amplitude of the pattern evoked major positive component is the most frequently used measurement parameter

b. The latency of the pattern evoked major positive component is usually in the region of 100 ms in normal adults

c. Optic nerve demyelination will give an increased amplitude, reduced latency pattern evoked major positive component

d. An amblyopic eye will usually have a normal flash visual evoked potential but an abnormal pattern visual evoked potential

e. Diseases of the eye do not produce an increase in pattern evoked major positive component latency

The pattern visual evoked potential to a reversing checkerboard contains a prominent positive component at approximately 100 ms (usually known as the P_{100} component). This is preceded and followed by negative components at approximately 70 and 135 ms respectively, known as N_{70} and N_{135}. The latency of the P_{100} component is the most frequently used measure, although amplitude can also be relevant. Optic nerve demyelination characteristically produces a delay in P_{100}, often associated with an amplitude reduction, the magnitude of the amplitude reduction being loosely correlated with the visual acuity. An amblyopic eye will give a normal flash visual evoked potential but an abnormal pattern visual evoked potential. Eye disease will often cause both an increase in latency and a reduction in amplitude of the P_{100} component. Nomenclature in the flash visual evoked potential is less uniformly accepted, but P1 is often used to describe the early positive component at approximately 70 ms and P2 for the major positive component at approximately 110 ms.

11.10 *Uses of the visual evoked potential*

a. Visual evoked potentials are useful in cases of functional visual loss
b. The pattern electroretinogram alone can distinguish between retinal and optic nerve disease
c. The pattern visual evoked potential may be used to give an approximate measure of visual acuity
d. A delayed pattern visual evoked potential is specific for optic nerve demyelination
e. Pattern visual evoked potentials in patients with chiasmal compression show no interhemispheric asymmetry with monocular stimulation

Normal flash and pattern visual evoked potentials in the presence of symptoms which strongly suggest otherwise are consistent with functional visual loss, but it should be remembered that normal electrophysiological findings do not preclude the existence of some underlying organic dysfunction. Combined use of the electroretinogram and the pattern electroretinogram are also necessary to exclude peripheral retinal dysfunction, and central retinal dysfunction. A rough estimate of visual acuity can be obtained using pattern stimuli with progressively smaller elements; a pattern onset stimulus, where the pattern appears from a uniform background with the same overall luminance, is most appropriate for this application. Even with pattern reversal stimulation it is unlikely that a normal pattern visual evoked potential would be obtained from an eye with a visual acuity of 6/36 or less. The pattern electroretinogram helps to interpret an abnormal pattern visual evoked potential. Macular disease will often give a delayed pattern visual evoked potential, but will almost invariably also give a very abnormal P_{50} component; the pattern electroretinogram is often normal in optic nerve disease. Latency delays frequently occur in diseases of the optic nerve other than demyelination. This is particularly true for compression but can also occur in ischaemic optic neuropathy and other optic nerve diseases. Due to the effects on the decussating fibres in the optic chiasm, monocular pattern visual evoked potentials will usually be markedly asymmetrical across the hemispheres in chiasmal compression, giving a "crossed" asymmetry where the findings from the two eyes show an opposite pattern of asymmetry.

12: **The visual pathways**

In the following section questions referring to the ultrastructure of the lateral geniculate nucleus are based on research carried out on higher primates such as the Rhesus monkey, as there is thought to be a close correlation between the geniculate ultrastructure in these primates and that in humans.

12.1 *Lateral geniculate nuclei*

a. The lateral geniculate nuclei
b. Each nucleus has six ventral layers and four dorsal layers
c. Their medial aspect receives information from the inferior visual field
d. Layers 2, 3 and 5 receive contralateral retinal fibres
e. The lateral geniculate nuclei receive fibres from the visual cortex

The lateral geniculate nuclei are paired thalamic nuclei in which the retinal ganglion cells synapse. They are retinotopically mapped with information from the superior retina and the inferior visual field relaying to the medial aspect of the nucleus. Layers 1 and 2 are magnocellular and layers 3–6 are parvocellular (layers 4 and 6 plus 3 and 5 fuse anteriorly, forming four ventral layers). Layers 2, 3 and 5 receive input from the ipsilateral eye. However, input is not restricted to ganglion cells and corticofugal fibres from the visual cortex synapse on geniculocortical cells and interneurones in the synaptic "glomeruli".

12.2 *Physiology of the lateral geniculate nucleus*

a. Receptive fields of lateral geniculate nucleus cells have "centre surround" organisation
b. Y cells respond optimally to temporally modulated stimuli
c. Colour coded cells are Y like cells
d. Colour coded cells are predominantly parvocellular
e. Cells terminate in layer III of the visual cortex

The receptive fields of the lateral geniculate nuclei cells have a centre surround organisation with "on/off" centres (demonstrated in monkey and cat lateral geniculate nuclei). The major cell types are x and y cells, the response properties of which are similar to the ganglion cells they connect with. Y cells respond optimally to temporally modulated stimuli and are therefore suited for temporal resolution. X cells respond maximally to static stimuli, and colour coded (parvocellular type) and are suited for spatial resolution. Both types synapse in the fourth layer of the visual cortex.

12.3 *The striate cortex*

a. The striate cortex is Brodman's area 17
b. The striate cortex is composed of five layers
c. Layer IV is the thickest layer
d. Pyramidal cells are predominantly found in layer IV
e. Stellate cells are predominantly found in layer VI

Gennari described the striate cortex in 1782 while still a medical student. It is found in the occipital cortex, Brodman's area 17. It has a six layered structure (as does all the cerebral cortex), but a feature unique to the visual cortex is a macroscopic stripe visible in layer IV, the stripe of Gennari. Layer IV is the thickest layer; it receives efferents from the lateral geniculate nucleus and contains predominantly stellate cells. The sixth layer sends efferents to the lateral geniculate nucleus and contains predominantly pyramidal cells.

12.4 *Physiology of the cortical cells*

a. Concentric cells have centre surround receptive fields
b. Simple cells are found mainly in layer IV
c. Complex cells respond best to a stimulus of a specific orientation moving in a specific direction
d. Complex cells receive binocular input and are rarely found in layer IV
e. Hypercomplex cells require the line stimulus to be of a specific length as well as a specific orientation and direction

273

The cortical cells and receptive field structure was established by Hubel and Wiesel, and from this they inferred a receptive field hierarchy. According to this model there are four types of visual cortical cells.

(1) Concentric cells, which have a centre surround receptive field.

(2) Simple cells: these are found mainly in layer IV and have receptive fields in simple parallel bands.

(3) Complex cells have a binocular input and are found on either side of layer IV (layers III and V). They respond to a stimulus of a specific orientation moving in a specific direction.

(4) Hypercomplex cells are more advanced in that the stimulus should also be of a specific length, so called "end inhibition".

However, this "model" has undergone some modifications in the light of recent research—for example, the phenomenon of "end inhibition", originally thought to be exclusive to hypercomplex cells, has been found in some simple cells.

12.5 *Synaptic connections*

a. Cortical geniculate cells synapse with retinogeniculate cells and interneurones
b. Layer V cells connect to the superior colliculus
c. The pulvinar and the extrastriate cortex are connected
d. Intercortical connections exist via the corpus callosum
e. Connections exist between the visual cortex and cerebellum

Cortical geniculate cells originate from layer VI of the visual cortex and synapse with ganglion cells and interneurones in the synaptic "glomeruli" of the lateral geniculate nucleus. Layer V cells relay to the superior colliculus whose connections with the medial longitudinal fasciculus enable ocular movements to be coordinated with "flashes" of light. The pulvinar is mainly connected to the extrastriate cortex but visual cortical connections do exist. Cells in layer II synapse with the contralateral visual cortex via the corpus callosum. This connection is not essential for binocular and stereoscopic vision as stereopsis is manifest at a cellular level in each hemisphere.

12.6 *Representation of the visual field on the visual cortex*

> a. The superior half of the visual field is represented below the calcarine sulcus
> b. The inferior half of the retina corresponds to the area above the calcarine sulcus
> c. No cortical lesion can produce a monocular defect
> d. The macula is represented at the anterior aspect of the calcarine sulcus
> e. Macular sparing is suggestive of a cortical lesion

The superior half of the visual field (and therefore the inferior half of the retina) correspond to the area below the calcarine sulcus. At the most anterior end of the sulcus is an area of cortex that corresponds solely to the most peripheral nasal retina: a lesion here will produce a defect in the "temporal crescent" of the contralateral eye only. The posterior end of the sulcus lies at the watershed region between the middle and posterior cerebral arteries, and the area of the cortex devoted to the macula is relatively large; these factors may account for the macular sparing seen in some cortical lesions.

12.7 *Visual deprivation in the perinatal period*

> a. Binocular stimulus deprivation hinders the development of neurones with an oriented receptive field
> b. Binocular stimulus deprivation inhibits the development of a binocular input to cortical cells
> c. Monocular stimulus deprivation causes loss of binocular input to cortical cells
> d. Monocular stimulus deprivation causes a change in cortical and lateral geniculate nucleus morphology
> e. Monocular stimulus deprivation predominantly affects Y type cells

Most of the research on the development and maturation of the visual pathways has been carried out on kittens, and young primates. In this work stimulus deprivation was achieved by a number of methods, including suturing of the eyelids and dark rearing. Binocular stimulus deprivation will prevent neurones developing oriented receptor fields, but binocularity *will* exist. Normal binocular development will, however, be disrupted by uniocular stimulus deprivation in the perinatal period, as this results in "competition" between the cortical afferents. Uniocular stimulus deprivation will produce a decrease in the size of lateral geniculate nucleus cells receiving input from that eye (mostly Y cells), and a change in the morphology of cortical layer IV which receives geniculate efferents.

12.8 *The "critical period" for acuity in humans*

a. The "critical period" begins at approximately 4 months
b. It is present up to 12 years
c. The severity of the visual deficit depends solely on the duration and degree of visual deprivation
d. The critical period for binocularity is longer than that for acuity
e. Amblyopia is often a result of monocular deprivation in the critical period

The exact details of the critical period in humans are not as well defined as those for experimental animals (cats and monkeys). It is thought to begin at 4 months and has a maximum sensitivity at 6–9 months. It then declines steadily until the age of 8 years. Amblyopia is a common sequela of stimulus deprivation. The degree of amblyopia is dependent not only on the degree and duration of the visual deprivation, but also on its timing. Even short periods of visual deprivation (as little as 3–4 days) between the ages of 6 and 18 months can result in profound amblyopia. The critical period for binocularity peaks at 1–3 years and decreases until the age of 6 years.

13: Visual acuity and adaptation

13.1 *Optotypes and Snellen letters*

a. 6/6 (20/20 or 1.0) vision with a Landholdt C corresponds to a gap in the letter which subtends (at the eye) 2.5 min of arc
b. 6/6 (20/20 or 1.0) vision with a Landholdt C corresponds to a gap in the letter which subtends (at the eye) 1.5 min of arc
c. 6/6 (20/20 or 1.0) vision with a Landholdt C corresponds to a gap in the letter which subtends (at the eye) 1.0 min of arc
d. 6/18 (20/60 or 0.33) vision with a Snellen letter corresponds to a letter height which subtends (at the eye) 3 min arc
e. 6/12 (20/40 or 0.5) vision with a Snellen chart corresponds to a letter height which subtends (at the eye) 10 min arc

Optotypes all derive from the Landholdt "C". The Snellen letters are made so that the gaps between letter elements are adjusted in size to correspond to 1 minute for the 6/6 letter. Other optotypes (e.g. the Sloan letters) use slightly different formulations. Spacing between the letters also affects visual performance. A recent international standard gives complete details.

13.2 *Measurement of spatial contrast sensitivity function*

The spatial contrast sensitivity function is measured with:
a. Chequerboards
b. Gey optotype letters
c. Ronchi gratings
d. Sinusoidal gratings
e. Stripes

13.3

In fig 101 the y axis represents the luminance of a grating, and the x axis distance across the grating, so the luminance varies sinusoidally. Light intensity is indicated at places by the symbols x, y, and z. The contrast of the grating is defined as:

a. $x - y$

b. x/y

c. $(x - y)/(x + y)$

d. x/z

e. y/z

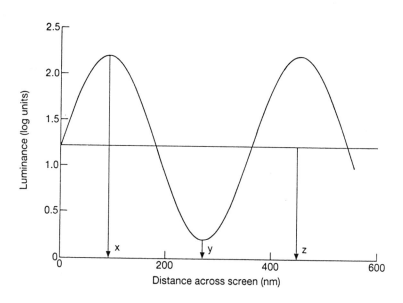

Fig 101 Luminance distribution in a sinusoidal grating

13.4

> The minimal value of contrast visible with sinusoidal gratings under optimal conditions varies with the spacing of the grating, defined as cycles/degree.
> a. The optimal value at normal illumination levels is 1 cycle/degree
> b. The optimal value at normal illumination levels is 3 cycles/degree
> c. The optimal value at normal illumination levels is 10 cycles/degree
> d. The minimum contrast detectable is 0.5%
> e. The minimum contrast detectable is 2.0%

For very small optotype letters contrast must be 100% before they are visible, but for larger objects recognition is possible with lower contrast – that is, the object need not be black on white, but grey on grey. The change in contrast threshold as a function of variation of the size of an object is an important variable but real objects are detected by border contrast. Therefore spatially sinusoidal gratings are commonly employed, since the gradient of luminance decreases as the width between successive bars increases. Other "grey" objects can be used, but the sharp edges of optotype letters introduce higher spatial frequencies. The contrast of the grating is defined as $(x - y)/(x + y)$. Measurement of low spatial frequencies with very large letters therefore gives ambiguous results. The minimum contrast visible for sinusoidal gratings is 0.5%. This optimum value is attained with spacings of 1 cycle/degree at normal illumination levels.

13.5 Vernier acuity

> In young adult emmetropes, free viewing, with optimum illumination.
> a. The minimum detectable visual angle of vernier is 10 arc sec
> b. Visual acuity is limited by the spacing of retinal receptors
> c. Diffraction of the pupil
> d. Optical interference within the cones
> e. Imperfections in the lens

The ability to detect breaks in lines, the vernier acuity, is much better than optotype acuity. The minimum detectable visual angle of the vernier is 1 arc sec. The spacing of retinal receptors was thought to be the limiting value for foveal acuity, and foveal midget ganglion cells are frequently connected to a single cone, via a single midget bipolar cell. The spacing between adjacent foveal cones approximates to 1' arc. However, the optical pathway contains many aberrations, and if the boundary of a black/white image (100% contrast) lies on a cone, the contrast difference from the adjacent foveal cone is about 1%, which limits the ability of the higher levels of the central nervous system to extract feature information. Therefore, if the optics of the eye are bypassed (e.g. by using lasers) visual acuity is always higher than when determined with natural optics, no matter what measure is used. In addition, the rate of quantal absorption at any illumination varies with the square root of the mean number of quanta. This imposes a theoretical minimum illumination difference for detection of edges and, for illuminations $< 10^5$ threshold acuity is limited by this cause. Many judgments can be made to greater precision than visual acuity. These are *hyperacuity* tasks. It is supposed that when an image of a border falls on a number of cones, the spatial relation between the array of photoreceptors can be interpreted by cortical mechanisms to achieve such precision.

13.6 *Pupil size and visual acuity*

Visual acuity can *improve* with decreasing pupillary apertures because:
a. The periphery of the lens is optically poor
b. Diffraction by the pupil increases retinal contrast
c. The size of the retinal image increases
d. The intraocular pressure drops
e. Of an increased Stiles-Crawford effect

13.7 *Decreasing pupil size*

Decreasing pupil size can *reduce* acuity because:
a. The luminance of the retinal image decreases
b. Diffraction by the iris decreases retinal contrast
c. Glare caused by lens nucleus reduces retinal contrast
d. The clear area of the lens is no longer in the optic axis
e. Chromatic aberration increases

The optimum pupillary aperture is a compromise between the reduction in retinal illumination as the pupil constricts, the decrease in refractive error associated with a small pupil, and the increase in diffraction causing loss of contrast. The optimal aperture is 2.8 mm.

13.8 *Visual acuity from the fovea to the periphery*

Visual acuity decreases from the fovea to the periphery because of:
a. Reduction in number of cones/unit area
b. Increase in area of bipolar cell dendritic expansions
c. Increase in size of ganglion cell receptive fields
d. Alteration in the cortical magnification factor
e. Irregular errors of refraction in the vitreous

Foveal midget ganglion cells contact a single cone. Peripheral midget ganglion cells are connected to as many as three or four cones. Cones lie among and are separated by rods, and the rod:cone ratio increases towards the periphery, so the area of the receptive field increases. The number of cortical cells per unit visual angle is probably the prime determinant of visual acuity because visual acuity falls more rapidly than the increase in the size of retinal units.

13.9 *Monochromats*

People who congenitally have no colour vision (monochromats):
a. May have visual acuity of 20/20
b. Usually have visual acuity <20/200
c. Have residual extrafoveal cones
d. Have blue cones
e. Are night blind

There are three classes of people who congenitally have no colour vision (monochromats). Very rarely, although foveal cones are normal, there is no colour discrimination but vision is otherwise normal. Usually the fovea is deficient in cones, so daylight vision is mediated through extrafoveal rods: the result is a gross reduction in visual acuity, photophobia and nystagmus. There may be some cones present in the periphery. A rare class of apparently monochromatic observers has vision between 0.1 and 0.3, no nystagmus and little or no photophobia. These people have normal blue cone function, and some colour discrimination in the blue region of the spectrum.

13.10 *Albinos*

Factors contributing to poor visual acuity in albinos include:
a. Lack of melanin pigment
b. Rods are found in the fovea
c. Cones are absent in the fovea
d. Optic nerve fibres make anomalous connections in the visual cortex
e. Nystagmus

While loss of melanin can contribute to glare, the poor visual acuity of albinos is related to anomalous insertion of retinal afferents in the cortex, and this is related to nystagmus. In all ocular albinos and in oculo-cutaneous albinos the fovea is poorly developed.

13.11 *Spectral sensitivity*

Photopic spectral sensitivity in the retinal periphery is relatively higher than in the fovea:
a. In the blue region of the spectrum
b. In the green region of the spectrum
c. In the red region of the spectrum
d. In the blue, green, and red regions of the spectrum
e. In none of these three regions

In the blue region of the spectrum, the sensitivity of the macula is depressed by the yellow macular pigment. In addition, the proportion of blue cones relative to the other cones rises from 0 at the central 20' (where blue cones are totally absent) to a maximum at 7–10°.

13.12 *Visual acuity in the newborn*

a. 6/6
b. 6/12
c. 6/36
d. 6/60
e. CF

Acuity in babies is determined by the techniques of preferential looking or measuring evoked potentials, and the latter give slightly higher results. Both methods agree that in the newborn stripes (gratings) of about 1 cycle/degree are the maximum resolvable – that is, one thirtieth of the adult level. Apart from the immature optical pathways, the neural connection of the retina and the visual cortex are not fully developed, and continue to differentiate until at least 8 years of age.

13.13 *Measurement of the temporal properties of vision*

Figure 102 represents the fluctuating (flickering) temporal output of a light source. If the period from t_1 to t_2 decreases from 5 seconds to 100 msec the light will change in the following ways:

a. Flicker will seem to increase
b. The light will appear brighter
c. The light will become dimmer
d. The subjective brightness will not alter
e. The light will appear pink

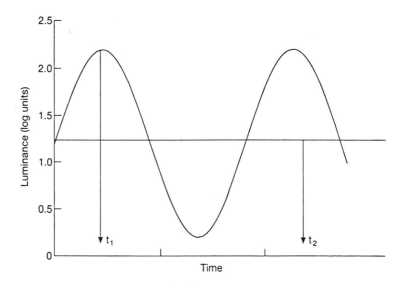

Fig 102 Temporal output of a flickering light source

13.14 *Persistance of a visual image*

> If the persistance of a visual image following a brief flash of
> light were to increase this would:
> a. Increase the flicker fusion rate
> b. Reduce the flicker fusion rate
> c. Leave the flicker fusion rate unchanged
> d. Alter colour sensation
> e. None of the above

The temporal properties of vision can be measured with a
sinusoidal flicker. For every temporal frequency, there is a
threshold contrast (compare with spatial contrast sensitivity in
section 13.2 above). Slowly varying light outputs cause adaptation to the new level of illumination, and are not noticeable
since the visual system in general only responds to a change in
light intensity. The optimal temporal frequency for perceiving
flicker is 10 Hz: at still higher frequencies the persistence of
excitation in photoreceptors becomes important, so that the
effective contrast of the flicker decreases. In addition, the
bipolar cells differentiate ("sharpen up") the signal, so lights
flickering at the optimal frequency appear brighter. Similarly,
there can be resonances in the brain which cause an apparent
increase in brightness. This phenomenon is known as the
Broca–Sulza effect.

13.15 *Critical frequency*

> The flicker of a temporally varying light source vanishes at a
> critical frequency. The frequency is affected by:
> a. The mean illumination
> b. The contrast
> c. The wavelength of flickering light
> d. The state of adaptation of the eye
> e. The presence of a pattern in the retinal image

The Ferry–Porter Law states that critical frequency varies with log mean luminance, and is true over large ranges of photopic illumination. De Lange's name is given to the *temporal* contrast sensitivity function which can be determined in a manner analogous to the *spatial* contrast sensitivity. For white light, minimum contrast is required for a 10 Hz flicker. Colour flicker can be used, and the "blue" or short wave mechanism responds more slowly and cuts off at lower temporal frequencies than does the red–green or black–white system.

13.16 *Properties of the scotopic system*

a. Rods respond only to single flashes
b. The maximum flicker rate perceptible is less than 10 Hz
c. Rods can signal flicker at > 20 Hz
d. Rods respond to lower flicker rates of red than blue light
e. Rod flicker fusion frequency decreases between the 10th and 30th minute of dark adaptation

Rods respond to very weak light only at low flicker rates. It can be shown that rods respond to more intense flashes of 30 Hz. If still higher intensities are used, the system saturates and only cone flicker signals can be transmitted. During dark adaptation scotopic sensitivity is initially very low (threshold high) and increases only slowly beyond cone sensitivity. Cone signals are inhibited by the rods, and flicker thresholds (and other thresholds) for red light rise. This can cause impairment of visual performance and can be seen, for example, when driving at night.

13.17 *Adaptation*

The visual threshold increases as the subject moves from absolute darkness to very bright sunlight by a factor of:
a. 14 log unit
b. 12 log unit
c. 10 log unit
d. 6 log unit
e. 3 log unit

13.18

Pupillary dilatation in dark adaptation can account for an increase of sensitivity of:
a. 0.5 log unit
b. 0.7 log unit
c. 1.3 log unit
d. 1.7 log unit
e. 2.5 log unit

13.19

Threshold of vision in the totally dark adapted eye corresponds to:
a. The absorption of a single quantum
b. 1 quantum absorbed in each of a number of adjacent rods
c. One in 10 rods absorbing a quantum
d. 3–10 quanta/degree visual angle/100 ms
e. 100 quanta incident at the cornea

13.20

The eye loses sensitivity (of the rod system) when absolute darkness is replaced by dim ambient illumination (the level found inside a cinema). This is caused by:
a. Bleaching of rhodopsin
b. Saturation of the receptor dark current
c. Reduction in cGMP in the outer limb in cGMP
d. Desensitisation at the receptor–bipolar synapse
e. Reduction of the calcium in rod outer limbs

The range of intensities over which the eye can function is about 1×10^{12}, though at any point within this range a change in intensity of only about 1000-fold can be distinguished. Therefore the working range for vision changes as the ambient illumination alters, and this is called adaptation. Retinal illumination is proportional to pupillary area. The diameter increases fourfold in dark adaptation – that is, an increase in area of 16-fold (1.3 log unit). The exact amount depends on the initial size of the pupil, and the extent to which it can dilate, which is reduced in elderly people. Thus the regulation of sensitivity by the pupil is very limited. The change of sensitivity with time in the dark is known as the dark adaptation curve. It is classically in two parts: an early rapid increase in cone sensitivity is followed by a delayed slower increase in rod sensitivity. At absolute threshold, 4–10 quanta absorbed in an area containing several thousand rods can produce a visual sensation. Very dim lights which do not provide 1 quantum absorbed/second/rod nevertheless cause depression of rod sensitivity, and therefore changes at or after the first rod synapse are connected with light adaptation. The mechanism of transduction alters when the rod is constantly absorbing quanta. The "gain" at the rod synapse also reduces. Other slower neurohormonal factors may also operate. In normal room lighting, 95% of the total rhodopsin remains unbleached. During the course of dark adaptation there is a rough relationship between the proportion of rhodopsin bleached and the logarithm of loss of sensitivity, but this is empirical and the precise theoretical significance remains unexplained.

13.21 *Rod sensitivity*

You can ensure that vision can be mediated only by rods by:
a. Exposing the eye to a very bright light for 15 minutes
b. Placing the subject in darkness for 30 minutes
c. Placing a red filter before the eye for 25 minutes
d. Placing a blue filter before the eye
e. Stimulating the peripheral retina only

13.22 *Cone sensitivity*

You can ensure that vision can be mediated only by cones by:
a. Using a rapidly flickering stimulus
b. Using deep red light in the dark adapted eye
c. Focusing the image on the fovea
d. Using very small images in the periphery
e. Superimposing the stimulus on a constant bright light

Although there are many more rods in the peripheral retina than cones, they do not send signals to the brain in the light adapted state. Because rods absorb long wave-length light, red filters should not be used as the only method of dark-adaptation. Cones can follow flickering stimuli at a greater rate than rods, but the rate must be more than 30 Hz to ensure that the flickering sensation is cone-driven. The central 30′ of the visual field is rod free, but if a small image is focused on the rod free zone in complete dark adaptation, light scattered on to the adjacent rods will be detected by the more sensitive scotopic system. Although a considerable proportion of the scotopic sensitivity is due to neurophysiological factors such as the convergence of many receptors on to one bipolar, the signals produced by single quantal absorptions in rods are up to 10 times larger than in cones, so no matter how small the retinal area stimulated, rod sensitivity is always higher than cone sensitivity. With larger stimuli (such as those used in most dark adaptometers) long flashes of red light are sensed by cones in the normal, fully dark adapted eye.

14: Colour vision

14.1 *Cones*

a. There are three classes of cone photoreceptor
b. There are four classes of cone photoreceptor
c. Long wavelength cones absorb maximally in the red region of the spectrum
d. Long wavelength cones absorb maximally in the orange region of the spectrum
e. Long wavelength cones absorb maximally in the yellow-green region of the spectrum

There are three types of cone, and this gives rise to the trichromacy of normal vision. However, the three classes (short wavelength, medium wavelength and long wavelength cones) do not span the spectrum equally and the long wavelength cones absorb maximally at about 560 nm, which to our eyes appears green. The sensation of "red" is thus due to the interaction between medium wavelength and long wavelength cones.

14.2 *Number of classes of congenital colour defectives*

a. Four
b. Five
c. Six
d. Seven
e. Eight

14.3 *Differences between a protanope and a protanomalous person*

a. Sex
b. Severity of condition
c. The colours they confuse
d. The relative brightness of the mid-spectral region
e. The protanope completely lacks one colour mechanism

Colour defectives can be dichromats (protanopes, deuteranopes or tritanopes) who have only two colour mechanisms (probably lack one class of cone). Anomalous trichromats (protanomalous, deuteranomalous, tritanomalous) have three classes of cone, but the pigments are abnormal. Thus the colour-matches such people make are different from normal, and also their colour discrimination is reduced to a variable extent. In addition there are rod monochromats and rare monochromats who have normal cones, but no colour discrimination at all. In addition, female carriers of abnormal genes coding for red or for green pigments may have two or more different functional, but slightly dissimilar cone pigments, so there may be more than eight classes of colour defectives.

14.4 *Incidence of congenital colour defects*

a. 1% the male population
b. 2% the male population
c. 4% the male population
d. 8% the general population
e. 12% none of the above

The genes for medium (green) and long (red) wavelength pigments are found on the X chromosome and are therefore inherited as X-linked recession traits. Five per cent of males are deuteranomalous and 1% are deuteranopes, protanopes, or protanomalous—that is, 8% of the male population have congenital colour defects. The gene for the short (blue) wavelength is found on chromosome 7. Tritanomalous and tritanopic defects are found on 0.0001% and 0.001% of the male population respectively and are inherited as autosomal dominant traits.

14.5 *Colour mechanisms damaged by optic nerve disease*

a. Protan
b. Deuteran
c. Tritan
d. All of the above
e. None of the above

Most retinal disease causes a disproportionate loss of tritan discrimination, but optic nerve disease affects all colour modalities.

15: Binocular vision and stereopsis

15.1 *Corresponding retinal points*

a. These are points which are the same angular distances from the foveal centre
b. Corresponding retinal points have zero binocular disparity
c. They are connected to approximately the same area of the visual cortex
d. A horopter is a curved line joining corresponding retinal points on the retina
e. Images must fall on corresponding retinal points to be perceived as single

Corresponding retinal points are the same angular distance from the two foveal centres. They have zero binocular disparity and are connected to approximately the same areas of the visual cortex. A horopter is a line in space connecting a set of points whose binocular disparity is zero. Numerous types of horopters have been described, including the geometric, empirical and distance horopters. Images found anywhere in Panum's area (a region bordering a horopter) will be perceived as single even if they fall on slightly non-corresponding retinal points.

15.2 *Requirements for binocular single vision*

a. Overlapping visual fields
b. Sensory fusion
c. Corresponding retinal elements
d. Normal stereopsis
e. Normally functioning extraocular muscles

Binocular single vision has a number of sensory aspects.

(1) Visual direction. This refers to a stimulus that falls on corresponding retinal points in two eyes and is therefore perceived as being in the same visual direction whichever eye views the stimulus. This will require normally functioning extraocular muscles if binocular single vision is to be

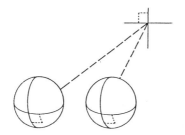

(a)

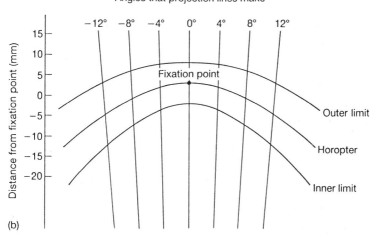

(b)

Fig 103 Binocular vision: (a) geometric retinal correspondence; (b) region of binocular single vision: Panum's area

attained in all positions of gaze. However, even patients with a paretic muscle (an isolated right sixth nerve palsy) will have some degree of binocular single vision in the left field of gaze

(2) Sensory fusion. Here images that have a slight binocular disparity, but fall inside Panum's area, will be perceived as single

(3) Dichoptic stimulation. If dissimilar images or contours are present in the same retinal area a binocular rivalry will develop

(4) Stereopsis. This may be defined as the ability to use binocular disparities to perceive distance in the third dimension of space. Stereopsis is not a prerequisite for binocular single vision.

15.3 *Diplopia*

a. Diplopia is a sensation produced by stimulating two points outside Panum's area
b. An uncrossed diplopia is produced by an image distant to the fixation point
c. A crossed diplopia is caused by stimulation of the nasal retina
d. Heterotropias are physiological diplopias
e. Exotropias cause an uncrossed diplopia

Diplopia may be defined as the sensation produced by stimulating two points outside Panum's area. Diplopias may be physiological or non-physiological (heterotropias). An uncrossed or homonymous diplopia is caused by the image of an object distant to the fixation site falling on the nasal retina. A crossed diplopia, which is found in exotropias, is caused by stimulation of the temporal retina.

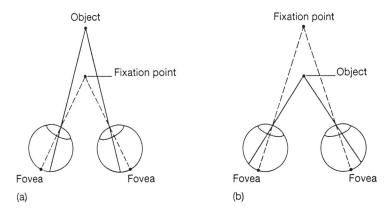

Fig 104 Diplopias: (a) uncrossed diplopia; (b) crossed diplopia

15.4 *Non-physiological diplopias*

a. There are three types of binocular diplopia
b. A heterotropia describes a latent deviation
c. The angle of a concomitant squint varies with the fixating eye and the direction of gaze
d. Primary deviation describes the deviation produced when the involved eye is fixating
e. In the acute situation the secondary deviation is less than the primary deviation

Heterotropias are manifest deviations and may be horizontal (esotropias, or exotropias), vertical, or tortional. Heterophorias are latent deviations. The size of a concomitant squint will not vary with the fixating eye or the direction of gaze, unlike that of an incomitant squint. The primary deviation describes the deviation seen in an incomitant squint when the uninvolved eye is fixating. In the acute situation this is always less than the secondary deviation, which is seen when the involved eye is fixating.

15.5 *Stereopsis*

> a. Stereopsis is possible without binocular single vision
> b. Stereopsis is poor beyond 20° from the fovea
> c. Disparities of 10″ are undetectable
> d. Stereopsis varies with object size
> e. Stereopsis may be measured by the Frisby test

Stereopsis is the ability to see an object in three dimensions. Binocular single vision is not a prerequisite for stereopsis: depth perception is possible even though retinal images are sufficiently disparate to be seen as double. The resolution of

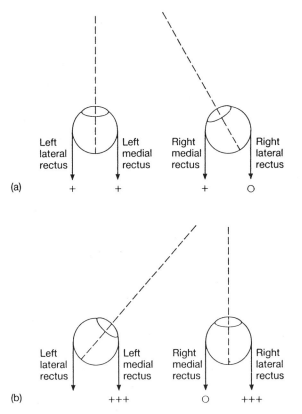

Fig 105 Right lateral rectus palsy: (a) primary deviation (fixation left eye); (b) secondary elevation (fixation right eye)

stereopsis enables disparities of 10″ (in some people 2″) or 0.0028° to be detected but is poor beyond 20° from the fovea and varies with object size. That is, disparity of a certain degree will be more easily detected in larger objects. Stereoacuity may be measured using three dimensional test objects or by haploscopic devices. In the latter test separate two dimensional targets are presented to each of the two eyes. The Frisby test employs random dot stereograms to achieve this effect.

Answers

1.1	a, e	**4.8**	a, b, c, d, e	**8.3**	a, c, d, e
1.2	c, d, e	**4.9**	a, c, d, e	**8.4**	a, b, c
1.3	a, b, d	**4.10**	b, c, e	**8.5**	b, d
1.4	a, c, d, e	**4.11**	b, e	**8.6**	a, b, c, d
1.5	a, c	**4.12**	d, e	**8.7**	b, d
1.6	a, b, c, d, e			**8.8**	b, c, d
		5.1	a, b	**8.9**	a, c, d
2.1	a, b, c, e	**5.2**	c, d, e	**8.10**	a, b, c
2.2	a, b, c, d	**5.3**	b, d, e	**8.11**	a, d, e
2.3	b, c, d, e	**5.4**	a, c, d, e	**8.12**	a, b, c
2.4	a, b, c, d	**5.5**	a, c, d, e	**8.13**	a, b, c, d
		5.6	c, d, e		
3.1	a, c, d, e	**5.7**	a, b, c, d, e	**9.1**	a, c, d
3.2	a, c, e			**9.2**	a, c, d, e
3.3	b, c, d, e	**6.1**	a, b	**9.3**	a, b, d, e
3.4	a, b, e	**6.2**	d, e	**9.4**	b, c, e
3.5	a, c, d, e	**6.3**	c, d, e	**9.5**	a, c, d
3.6	a, c, d, e	**6.4**	a, b, c, d, e	**9.6**	a, c, d
3.7	a, c, d	**6.5**	c, d	**9.7**	b, d
3.8	b, c, d	**6.6**	b, c, d, e	**9.8**	a, c
3.9	b, d			**9.9**	a, b, c, d, e
		7.1	a, d, e	**9.10**	c
4.1	a, b, c	**7.2**	a, b, c, d	**9.11**	a, c, d
4.2	b, c	**7.3**	a, c, e	**9.12**	a, c, d, e
4.3	a, b, c, d, e	**7.4**	a, b	**9.13**	a, c
4.4	c, d	**7.5**	a, b, c, e		
4.5	a, c, d			**10.1**	a, c, d
4.6	b, c, d	**8.1**	a, c, e	**10.2**	a, b, e
4.7	b, d, e	**8.2**	b, c, e	**10.3**	a, b, c, d

10.4	b, c, d, e	**11.10**	a, c	**13.12**	e
10.5	a, b, c			**13.13**	a, b
10.6	a, b, c, d	**12.1**	a, c, e	**13.14**	b
10.7	a, b, e	**12.2**	a, b, d	**13.15**	a, b, c, d
10.8	a, b, c, d, e	**12.3**	a, c	**13.16**	c
10.9	a, b, d, e	**12.4**	a, c, d, e	**13.17**	b
10.10	a, b, c, e	**12.5**	a, b, c, d	**13.18**	c, d
10.11	a, b, c, d	**12.6**	a, e	**13.19**	d, e
10.12	a, b, c, d	**12.7**	a, c, d, e	**13.20**	d
10.13	a, b, d, e	**12.8**	a, e	**13.21**	b
10.14	a, c, e			**13.22**	a, b, e
10.15	b, c, e	**13.1**	c, e		
		13.2	d	**14.1**	a, e
11.1	a, b, d	**13.3**	c	**14.2**	e
11.2	a, c, d	**13.4**	a, d	**14.3**	b, e
11.3	b, c	**13.5**	b, c, e	**14.4**	d
11.4	a, b, d	**13.6**	a	**14.5**	d
11.5	a, d	**13.7**	a, b		
11.6	a, b	**13.8**	a, b, c, d	**15.1**	a, b, c
11.7	b, c, e	**13.9**	a, b, c, d	**15.2**	a, b, c
11.8	a, e	**13.10**	a, c, d, e	**15.3**	a, b
11.9	b, d	**13.11**	a	**15.4**	a
				15.5	a, b, d, e

General physiology

1: Cardiovascular physiology

1.1 *Blood vessels*

> a. The aorta and large arteries are responsible for the Wind-kessel effect
> b. Arterioles have the maximum resistance to blood flow
> c. The total cross sectional area of the body's capillary beds is approximately 300 m^2
> d. Most of the blood volume is found in capillaries
> e. The velocity of blood flow in the venules is faster than in the vena cava

The aorta and other large arteries produce the Windkessel effect (the conversion of the intermittent blood flow in the aortic arch to a smooth axial flow). Arterioles are responsible for 50% of the peripheral vascular resistance. Capillaries have a surface area of approximately 300 m^2 but most (65%) of the blood volume is found in the veins and venules. The velocity of blood flow is greater in the vena cava than in the venules, because the cross sectional area of the vena cava is less than the total cross sectional area of the venules. The action of the "thoracic pump" will also contribute to this increased velocity.

1.2 *Autoregulation of blood flow*

> a. Myogenic regulation is present in the blood vessels of the lungs
> b. Oxygen deficiency causes vasodilatation in all tissues
> c. Increased CO_2 or H^+ concentration will promote an increase in blood flow
> d. Endothelial factors influence local blood flow
> e. Autoregulation is the main controlling influence on coronary blood flow

Autoregulation is designed either to keep the blood flow constant in the face of changing blood pressure or to adapt the blood flow to the needs of the local metabolism. The mechanisms of autoregulation are myogenic or metabolic. In the former mechanism a rise in blood pressure causing a dilatation will trigger a reflex vasoconstriction; however, this will not occur in the pulmonary arterioles. In metabolic autoregulation (which is the main influence on coronary blood flow) a decreased oxygen concentration, decreased pH, or raised CO_2 will cause vasodilatation and hence increase blood flow. This does not occur in the lungs, where a decrease in oxygen concentration causes vasoconstriction. Endothelial factors, such as endothelin (vasoconstriction), and nitric oxide (also known as endothelium-derived relaxing factor—vasodilatation) may have a marked effect on local blood flow.

1.3 Physics of flow in blood vessels

a. The velocity of flow in a vessel is inversely proportional to the cross sectional area of that vessel
b. Flow rate of blood in a vessel is proportional to the pressure difference along that vessel
c. The resistance of a vessel is inversely proportional to the fourth power of its radius
d. The resistance to flow in a vessel is proportional to the viscosity of the blood
e. The transmural pressure in a vessel (PT) equals the wall tension in the vessel (T) multiplied by the radius of the vessel

The velocity of fluid movement at any point in a system of tubes is inversely proportional to the *total* cross sectional area at that point. Therefore the average velocity of blood flow is high in the aorta, which has a small total cross sectional area, and low in the capillaries, which have a much larger total cross sectional area. The flow rate in a vessel is proportional to the pressure difference along that vessel. This is a modification of Ohm's law. The Poiseuille Hagen law states

$$R = 8L\eta/\pi r^4$$

where: R = resistance to flow; L = length of the vessel; r = the radius of the vessel; and η = viscosity of the blood.
La Place's law states that

$$T = PT \times R.$$

1.4 Neuronal control of circulation in blood vessels

a. Stimulation of α receptors causes vasoconstriction
b. Vasodilatation is caused by β_1 receptor stimulation
c. When metabolic and neuronal signals conflict, the metabolic ones take priority
d. α and β receptors are found in veins
e. Parasympathetic vasodilatation occurs in the vessels of sweat and salivary glands

Neuronal control of blood vessels is mediated with only a few exceptions by the sympathetic nerves. Postganglionic transmission involves α_1 receptors and causes vasoconstriction, whereas vasodilatation is produced by β_2 stimulation. Metabolic signals (such as raised CO_2 or lowered oxygen concentration) will override neuronal signalling. The α and β receptors in the venous system allow for the regulation of venous return to the heart. Sweat and salivary glands are the exception, mentioned above because parasympathetic stimulation will produce vasodilatation.

1.5 *Hormonal control of circulation in blood vessels*

> a. Noradrenaline produces only vasoconstriction
> b. Adrenaline has a vasodilatory effect in low concentrations
> c. Angiotensin II is a potent vasoconstrictor
> d. Histamine causes a pronounced vasoconstriction
> c. Bradykinin causes vasodilatation

Noradrenaline, which acts via α receptors, will produce only vasoconstriction. However, low concentrations of adrenaline will stimulate β_2 receptors, causing vasodilatation. Angiotensin II, as well as being one of the most potent vasoconstrictors, will stimulate thirst and production of aldosterone. Histamine and bradykinin produce vasodilatation of differing durations.

1.6 *Transcapillary exchange*

> Increased tissue fluid accumulation may be produced by:
> a. Increased arteriolar pressure
> b. Decreased venous pressure
> c. Decreased plasma oncotic pressure
> d. Increased capillary permeability
> e. Blockage of lymphatic drainage

The Starling hypothesis describes the driving forces responsible for filtration and reabsorption at the capillary wall. Increased pressure at the arterial end of the capillary bed will cause increased production of tissue fluid. Raised venous pressure decreases the absorption of tissue fluid. Similarly, a drop in plasma oncotic pressure (hypoproteinaemia) will cause increased accumulation of tissue fluid. Mediators of acute inflammation (such as histamine and endotoxins) may increase the permeability of capillaries and so increase oedema. Excess tissue fluid is normally drained via the lymphatics and so lymphatic blockage will predispose to oedema.

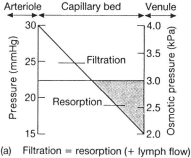

(a)   Filtration = resorption (+ lymph flow)

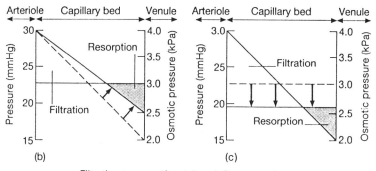

(b)

(c)

Filtration > resorption + lymph flow → oedema

Fig 106 Capillary fluid exchange

1.7 *Control of blood pressure*

a. Blood pressure = (heart rate × stroke volume) × peripheral resistance

b. Stimulation of aortic baroreceptors causes a bradycardia via the vagus nerve

c. Carotid baroreceptors are stimulated by a decrease in blood pressure

d. Stimulation of the aortic baroreceptors results in decreased vagal tone

e. The ocular cardiac reflex produces marked bradycardia

GENERAL PHYSIOLOGY

These two simple equations summarise how any drug can affect the blood pressure:

Blood pressure = cardiac output × peripheral resistance
Cardiac output = heart rate × stroke volume

Baroreceptors are specialised stretch receptors located in the aortic arch and carotid sinuses; they are stimulated by an increase in blood pressure and cause a reflex bradycardia. The aortic baroreceptors act via the vagus (increasing vagal tone) and the carotid via the glossopharyngeal nerves. The oculocardiac reflex will produce a bradycardia.

1.8 Starling's law

a. Increased venous return causes an increase in stroke volume
b. Increased venous return may have a positive chronotropic effect
c. Increased afterload initially causes a decrease in the stroke volume
d. Cardiac output continues to rise with increasing preload
e. An increase in contractility may cause an increase in stroke volume

Starling's law states that the force of a muscle contraction is proportional to the initial length of that muscle. An increase in venous return or preload will increase the stretching of the myocardium and cause an increase in stroke volume: a positive inotropic effect. It may also produce a positive chronotropic response by stimulating receptors at the venoatrial junctions. This is known as the Bainbridge reflex. However, if the preload continues to increase the stroke volume will eventually fall: this is congestive cardiac failure. An increase in peripheral resistance or afterload will initially cause the stroke volume to fall as the heart works against this increased resistance but will then result in an increased diastolic volume which increases the stretching of the myocardium and causes the stroke volume to rise. Inotropic drugs will increase the contractility of the myocardium, increasing stroke volume and cardiac output.

304

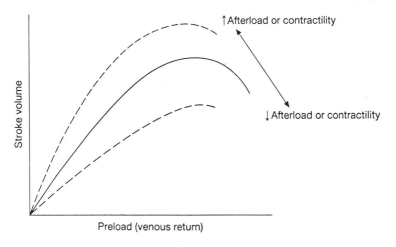

Fig 107 The Starling curve

2: Respiratory physiology

2.1 *Oxygen dissociation of haemoglobin*

a. The oxygen dissociation curve is a sigmoid curve
b. Increased P_{CO_2} causes a shift to the right
c. Increased temperature causes a shift to the left
d. An increase in pH causes a shift to the right
e. The percentage oxygen saturation of mixed venous blood (P_{VO_2} 40 mmHg) is about 75%

The oxygen dissociation curve of haemoglobin is a sigmoid curve. This is because of the "cooperative binding" of oxygen by haemoglobin (as haemoglobin takes up oxygen there is a change in the position of the haem moieties that favours further oxygen binding). The curve is shifted to the right (haemoglobin more readily gives up its bound oxygen) if CO_2 levels and temperature increase or if the pH is decreased. Under normal conditions the body operates near the plateau of the oxygen dissociation curve, which is why even mixed venous blood has an oxygen saturation of 75%.

305

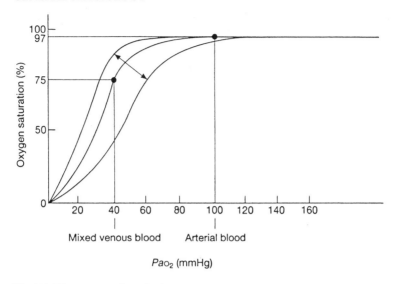

Fig 108 The oxygen dissociation curve of haemoglobin

2.2 Oxygen binding proteins

a. The fetal haemoglobin oxygen dissociation curve lies to the right of that in the adult
b. The oxygen dissociation curve of myoglobin lies to the left of that of haemoglobin in the adult
c. The carbon monoxide dissociation curve is much steeper than that of oxygen
d. Methaemoglobin has no affinity for oxygen
e. Anaemia changes the percentage oxygen saturation of the blood

The curve for fetal haemoglobin lies to the left of adult haemoglobin, that is, fetal haemoglobin has a higher affinity for oxygen. The curve for myoglobin also lies to the left of haemoglobin, which means it will give up its oxygen only in relatively hypoxic conditions such as in exercising muscle. Carbon monoxide has a very steep dissociation curve and even in small quantities will displace large amounts of oxygen from haemoglobin. Methaemoglobin is formed when ferrous iron is oxidised to ferric iron. It has no affinity for oxygen. Anaemia will decrease the total amount of oxygen carried but will not affect the percentage saturation.

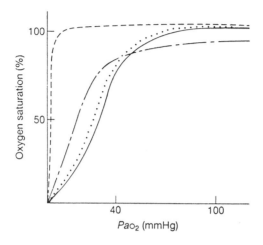

Fig 109 Oxygen binding curves: — haemoglobin; .... fetal haemoglobin; --- carboxyhaemoglobin; — · — · myoblobin

2.3 Respiration

a. The tidal volume in an adult is approximately 0.5 litres
b. The vital capacity is the maximum volume expired after the deepest possible inspiration
c. The total lung volume minus the vital capacity equals the tidal volume
d. $FEV_1/FVC = 0.8$ in a young person
e. The FEV_1/FVC ratio increases in asthma

The average tidal volume in an adult is 500 ml. The vital capacity is the volume expired after the deepest possible inspiration. When this is subtracted from the total lung volume the remainder equals the residual volume, which is approximately

1.5 litres. The ratio of FEV_1 (forced inspiratory volume in 1 second) to FVC (forced vital capacity) is approximately 0.8 in a normal adult. This ratio will decrease in asthma but is unchanged in restrictive lung diseases, such as fibrosing alveolitis.

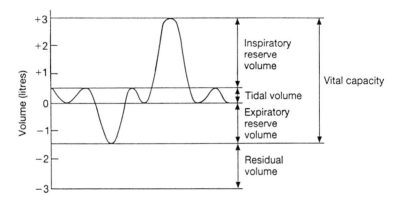

Fig 110 Lung volumes

2.4 *Ventilation: perfusion ratios*

a. Ventilation ($\dot{V}$) increases towards the base of the lungs (in the upright position)
b. Perfusion (Q) increases towards the base of the lungs (in the upright position)
c. The $\dot{V}$:Q ratio increases towards the base of the lungs (in the upright position)
d. The average alveolar Po_2 is 100 mmHg (13.3 kPa)
e. The pressure across the pulmonary capillary bed is approximately 35–25 mmHg

The ventilation of the alveoli increases towards the base of the lungs. However, perfusion of the capillary beds will increase to a greater extent and therefore the $\dot{V}$:Q ratio will decrease towards the base of the lungs. The normal alveolar Po_2 is

100 mmHg and the $P\text{co}_2$ is 40 mmHg. The pulmonary circulation is a low pressure circulation, with pressures across a pulmonary capillary bed of approximately 8 mmHg.

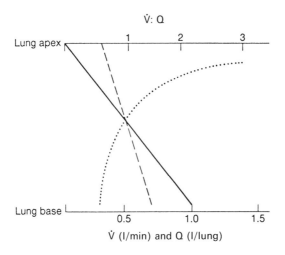

Fig 111 **Perfusion and ventilation of the lung.** —Q; - - - V̇; ......V̇:Q

3: Endocrinology

3.1 *Thyroid*

a. Thyroid stimulating hormone is a peptide hormone
b. Iodine ions are actively transported into the gland
c. Thyroglobulin is stored in follicular cells
d. Iodinated tyrosines couple to produce T3 and T4
e. Lysosomal enzymes are instrumental in cleaving hormones from thyroglobulin

Thyroid stimulating hormone is a glycoprotein hormone, produced by the anterior pituitary, which increases the active transport of iodine ions into the follicular cells. It will also increase thyroglobulin production and the coupling of iodinated tyrosines to produce triiodothyronine (T3) and thyroxine (T4). Thyroglobulin is synthesised in the rough endoplasmic reticulum and Golgi apparatus of the follicular cells but is stored in the colloid. Lysosomal enzymes will cleave T3 and T4 from thyroglobulin before they are released into the circulation.

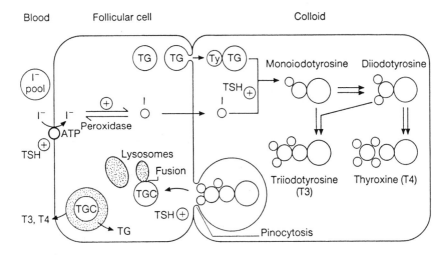

Fig 112 Production of thyroid hormone. TG, Thyroglobulin; TGC, thyroglobulin complex

3.2 Properties and functions of thyroid hormones

a. 99% of T3 and T4 is bound to albumin
b. T4 is two to three times as potent as T3
c. 80% of circulating T3 is derived from deiodinated T4
d. Thyroxines increase oxygen consumption in all tissues
e. T3 and T4 are needed for the conversion of carotenes to vitamin A in the liver

The ratio of T3 to T4 in the circulation is 1:100. Approximately 99% of these hormones in the circulation is bound to three different proteins: 80% to thyroid binding globulin, the remainder to thyroid binding prealbumin, and to albumin. Triiodothyronine is two or three times as potent as thyroxine. Of the circulating T3 80% is derived from deiodinated T4, not produced directly from the thyroid gland. The thyroid hormones increase the metabolic activity of most tissues by increasing the oxygen consumption. However, they will decrease the oxygen consumption of the anterior pituitary, aiding the negative feedback loop for production of thyroid stimulating hormone. Conversion of carotenes to vitamin A is facilitated by the thyroid hormones.

3.3 *Insulin production*

a. Insulin is produced by α cells in the islets of Langerhans
b. Insulin is a peptide hormone
c. Production of insulin is stimulated by increased blood glucose or amino acids
d. Production of insulin is stimulated by glucagon
e. Release of insulin is inhibited by β blockers

Insulin is an anabolic peptide hormone produced by the β cells of the islets of Langerhans in the pancreas. Its main role is in carbohydrate homoeostasis and its production is stimulated by increasing blood glucose, amino acids or glucagon. β Blockers will inhibit insulin release and their use should be avoided in diabetic patients, as they can also mask the warning signs of hypoglycaemia.

3.4 *Properties of insulin*

a. Increases glucose uptake into all cells
b. Increases glycogen production
c. Stimulates Na^+/K^+ ATPase pumps
d. Stimulates lipolysis
e. Inhibits glucagon release

Insulin increases the uptake of glucose into most tissues by increasing the number and activity of glucose transporting proteins in cell membranes. The brain and the retina are exceptions to this. The actions of insulin are anabolic, so it will promote glycogen production and inhibit lipolysis, gluconeo-genesis and glucagon production. The activity of the Na^+/K^+ ATPase pump is increased by insulin, which explains why potassium supplementation is required when treating diabetic ketoacidosis.

3.5 *Features of insulin deficiency*

> a. Osmotic diuresis
> b. Plasma hyperosmolarity
> c. Acidosis
> d. A negative nitrogen balance
> e. Increased glucagon concentrations

Poor control of insulin dependent diabetes mellitus may result in diabetic ketoacidosis. The symptoms and biochemical upsets seen in this condition are as much due to increased glucagon concentrations as they are to insulin deficiency. The triad of an osmotic diuresis (secondary to glycosuria), plasma hyperosmo-larity, and acidosis (secondary to ketones) is classically found in diabetic ketoacidosis.

3.6 *Production and functions of glucagon*

> a. Glucagon is produced by the β cells of the islets of Langerhans
> b. Glucagon decreases glycogenolysis
> c. Glucagon increases deamination of amino acids in the liver
> d. Blood levels of glucagon are increased by stress
> e. Production of glucagon is stimulated by insulin

Glucagon is a peptide hormone produced by the α cells of the islets of Langerhans. It is a catabolic hormone whose levels will be increased by "stress" (exercise, fright, and flight). Glucagon promotes glycogenolysis and the deamination of amino acids in the liver, which is often the initial step in gluconeogenesis. Insulin is a more powerful hormone than glucagon and will inhibit its production.

3.7 *Production of corticosteroids*

> a. Corticosteroids are produced in the zona glomerulosa
> b. The major precursor for corticosteroids is cholesterol
> c. Production is regulated by ACTH, which acts via cyclic AMP
> d. Most corticosteroids are unbound in the plasma
> e. Breakdown of corticosteroids occurs mainly in the liver

Mineralocorticoids are produced in the zona glomerulosa and corticosteroids in the zona fasciculata and reticularis of the adrenal cortex. Cholesterol is the main precursor for corticosteroid hormones, whose production is controlled by adrenocorticotrophic hormone (ACTH). This is a peptide hormone produced by the anterior pituitary, whose secondary messenger is cyclic AMP. Circulating corticosteroids are bound to transcortin (a specific binding protein) or albumin and are mainly metabolised in the liver by conjugation with sulphates or glucuronic acid.

3.8 *Effects of corticosteroids*

> a. Metabolic effects are generally anabolic
> b. Corticosteroids inhibit glucose uptake in most tissues
> c. Corticosteroids potentiate the pressor and bronchodilator effects of catecholamines
> d. Corticosteroids decrease protein breakdown
> e. Corticosteroids inhibit fibroblasts

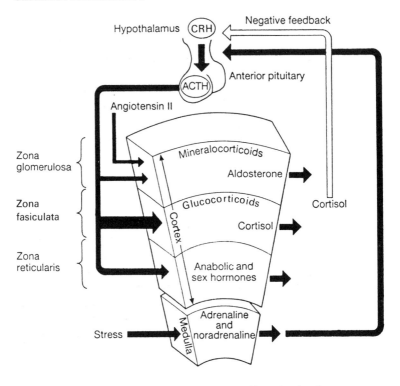

Fig 113 The adrenal gland. CRH, Corticotrophin releasing hormone

Corticosteroid secretion follows a diurnal pattern, with a peak at 0600 and a trough at 2400. They have a myriad of actions, which include

(1) Raising blood glucose by inhibiting glucose uptake into most tissues

(2) Potentiation of the effects of catecholamines on the circulation and in the lungs

(3) Stimulating catabolism of proteins, which may cause myopathies and the striae seen in Cushing's syndrome

(4) Inhibiting fibroblasts, so impeding wound healing.

3.9 *The adrenal medulla*

a. The ratio of adrenaline to noradrenaline in the adrenal medulla is approximately 1:6
b. Opioid peptides are also produced by the medulla
c. Phenylethanolamine-*N*-methyltransferase is unique to the medulla and central nervous system
d. Preganglionic sympathetic neurones synapse on cells of the medulla
e. Hypoglycaemia stimulates the medulla

The adrenal medulla is a neuroendocrine transducer in which neuronal impulses from preganglionic sympathetic nerves are converted into hormonal signals. Phenylethanolamine-*N*-methyltransferase is found only in the medulla and central nervous system and is responsible for the conversion of noradrenaline to adrenaline. The ratio of noradrenaline to adrenaline in the medulla is 1:6. Opioid peptides are also produced by the medulla. The classical symptoms and signs of hypoglycaemia are in the main attributable to an increase in catecholamines, and may be "masked" by beta blockers.

3.10 *Properties of catecholamines*

a. Adrenaline causes a decrease in circulatory resistance
b. Noradrenaline causes an increase in circulatory resistance
c. Adrenaline and noradrenaline cause bronchodilatation
d. The half life of adrenaline in the circulation is approximately 10 min
e. Most catecholamines are converted to vanillylmandelic acid in the liver

Catecholamines have differing cardiovascular actions. Adrenaline will produce a vasodilatation (via β_2 receptors) in skeletal muscle and liver blood vessels that exceeds its vasoconstrictive effects elsewhere, so decreasing total peripheral resistance. Noradrenaline, which has no vasodilatory effects, will increase circulatory resistance, so increasing the blood pressure. This stimulates the baroreceptor reflex which decreases cardiac output. Adrenaline is used to treat bronchospasm because of its β_2 agonist properties (noradrenaline also produces bronchodilatation). The half life of catecholamines in the circulation is approximately 2 min. About 50% of catecholamines are methoxylated and excreted, 30% being converted to vanillylmandelic acid.

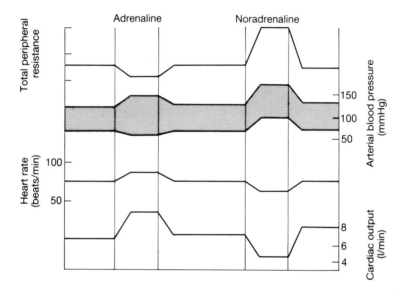

Fig 114 Circulatory effects of catecholamines

3.11 *Pituitary hormones*

a. Follicle stimulating hormone and luteinising hormone are produced by the anterior pituitary
b. Antidiuretic hormone and oxytocin are produced by the cells of the posterior pituitary
c. Prolactin production is increased by thyrotrophin releasing hormone
d. Adrenocorticotrophin and growth hormone are produced by the anterior pituitary
e. Hormones from the posterior pituitary are released into the systemic circulation

The pituitary gland is divided into two separate glands. The anterior pituitary (or adenohypophysis) produces follicle stimulating hormone, luteinising hormone, thyroid stimulating hormone, adrenocorticotrophin growth hormone, STH, and prolactin (whose release is stimulated by thyrotrophin releasing hormone). The posterior pituitary (neurohypophysis) is intimately connected with hypothalamic nuclei: antidiuretic hormone and oxytocin are produced in these nuclei and travel down axons by axoplasmic flow to the posterior pituitary. Here they are released directly into the systemic circulation, unlike anterior pituitary hormones, which are released into the portal hypophyseal circulation.

4: Renal physiology

4.1 *Functions of the kidney*

a. Acid–base regulation
b. Erythropoietin production
c. Prostaglandin and kinin production
d. Hydroxylation of 1-hydroxycholecalciferol
e. Maintenance of the correct concentration of all ions in the interstitial fluid

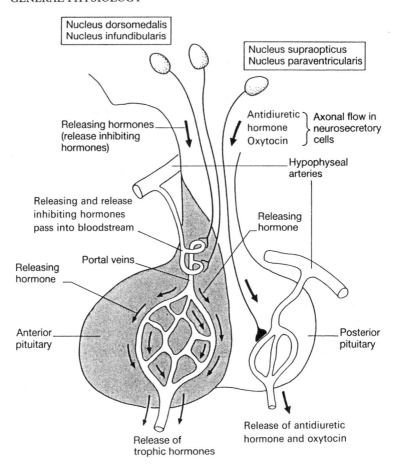

Nucleus dorsomedalis
Nucleus infundibularis

Nucleus supraopticus
Nucleus paraventricularis

Releasing hormones
(release inhibiting
hormones)

Antidiuretic ⎤ Axonal flow in
hormone ⎬ neurosecretory
Oxytocin ⎦ cells

Hypophyseal
arteries

Releasing and release
inhibiting hormones
pass into bloodstream

Releasing
hormone

Portal veins

Releasing
hormone

Releasing
hormone

Anterior
pituitary

Posterior
pituitary

Release of
trophic hormones

Release of antidiuretic
hormone and oxytocin

Fig 115 The hypothalamic-pituitary system

The kidney's most vital functions are the maintenance of the correct interstitial fluid ion concentrations, and the excretion of the waste products of metabolism. The kidneys play an integral part in acid–base balance by regulating bicarbonate production in their tubular cells. The anaemia of patients with chronic renal failure is due to a deficiency in erythropoietin, which is produced by the kidneys. The role of the kidney in vitamin D metabolism is to hydroxylate 25-hydroxycholecalciferol to 1,25-dihydroxycholecalciferol. Prostaglandins and kinins are also produced by the kidneys.

318

4.2 Glomerular filtration

a. Rate of glomerular filtration is approximately 250 ml/min
b. Glomerular filtration is partly dependent on the hydrostatic pressure in the glomerular capillaries
c. The glomerular filtration rate may be varied by the action of mesangial cells
d. Anions pass more freely into the filtrate than cations
e. Autoregulation of the glomerular capillary pressure occurs

The glomerular filtration rate is the volume filtered by all the glomeruli per unit time. An average of 20% of the renal plasma flow is filtered, producing a rate of 120 ml/min. The forces governing glomerular filtration are the same as those described by Starling for any capillary bed. One of these variables is the blood pressure in the glomerular capillaries, which may be autoregulated. This explains why the glomerular filtration rate will remain constant over a wide range of blood pressures. Mesangial cells found at the bifurcations of capillary loops have contractile properties which enable them to alter the area available for filtration. The endothelium of the glomerular capillaries carries a negative charge, therefore anions pass less readily into the filtrate than cations.

4.3 Function of the renal tubules

a. Tubules reabsorb a constant amount of the sodium filtered
b. 80% of the filtered sodium is reabsorbed
c. Glucose is reabsorbed in the proximal tubule by secondary active transport
d. Water absorption is decreased by antidiuretic hormone
e. Potassium is actively reabsorbed from proximal, and secreted from distal, tubules

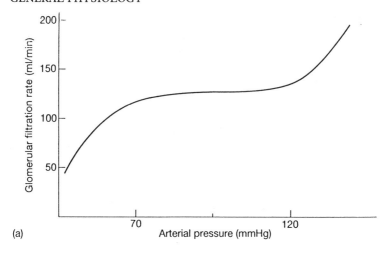

Fig 116 (a) Autoregulation of the glomerular filtration rate

The renal tubules reabsorb a constant *fraction* of the sodium filtered, not a constant *amount*—this is known as glomerulotubular balance. In the renal tubules 95–99.5% of filtered sodium is actively reabsorbed. In the proximal tubules much of this resorption is closely coupled with the cotransport of glucose and amino acids (known as secondary active transport). Antidiuretic hormone will increase the permeability of collecting ducts to water, thus increasing water reabsorption. Potassium is reabsorbed both passively and actively in the proximal tubules and is secreted under the influence of aldosterone in the distal tubules.

4.4 *Body water and osmolarity*

a. 60% of total body water is intracellular
b. 80% of the extracellular water is intravascular
c. Osmolality = mosmol/kg of solvent
d. Plasma proteins account for 90% of plasma osmolality
e. The difference in sodium concentration is the main determinant of fluid distribution across the capillary walls

320

Most (60%) of the total body water is intracellular; 40% is extracellular. Intravascular water accounts for only 20% of extracellular water. The osmolality of plasma is what determines the osmotic pressure of plasma and is measured in mosmol/kg of solvent. Sodium accounts for 90% of plasma osmolality but the sodium concentrations in the intravascular and extravascular compartments are approximately the same and therefore do not influence water movement across capillary walls. Plasma proteins produce an oncotic pressure which will, along with hydrostatic pressure, determine interstitial fluid production.

4.5 *Extracellular isotonic volume depletion of 500–1000 ml will cause*

   a. An increase in angiotensin II
   b. An increase in antidiuretic hormone
   c. Decreased aldosterone levels
   d. Increased sodium retention by the kidneys
   e. Thirst

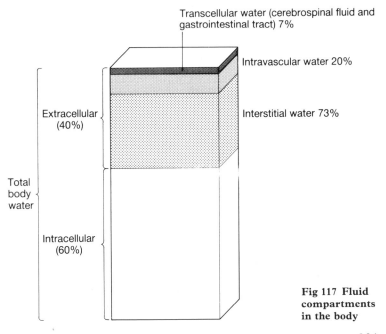

Transcellular water (cerebrospinal fluid and gastrointestinal tract) 7%

Intravascular water 20%

Extracellular (40%)

Interstitial water 73%

Total body water

Intracellular (60%)

Fig 117 Fluid compartments in the body

321

An isotonic loss of 500–1000 ml (such as in heavy bleeding) would be sufficient to stimulate the renin–angiotensin system. Angiotensin II is the final product of this pathway and directly stimulates aldosterone release and the thirst mechanism as well as causing vasoconstriction. Aldosterone will increase sodium reabsorption, an effect that takes approximately 1 hour and peaks at 4 hours. Antidiuretic hormone is released when hypertonic plasma stimulates hypothalamic osmoreceptors. An isotonic volume depletion of this magnitude will increase the production of this hormone by stimulation of volume receptors in the left atrium.

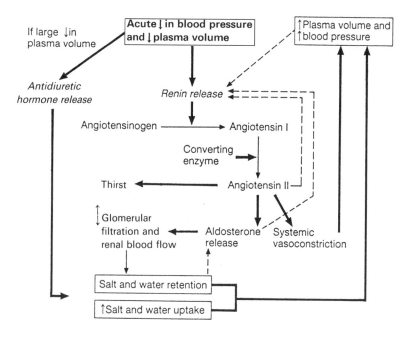

Fig 118 Homoeostatic response to isotonic volume depletion. ➡ Stimulatory action; --▶ inhibitory action

4.6 *Hypotonic fluid loss occurs in*

a. Excess sweating
b. Gastric losses
c. Patients with burns
d. Haemorrhage
e. The comatose patient

Sweat and gastric secretions are all hypotonic relative to plasma. Burns patients will suffer hypotonic losses because of the increased rate of evaporation from the damaged skin. The comatose patient, who may be ventilated, pyrexial and sweating, and unable to drink to replace losses will have an increased risk of hypotonic volume depletion. Isotonic losses are seen in haemorrhage or in biliary leaks.

4.7 *Causes and effects of acidosis*

a. Acidosis is caused by a fall in the $[HCO_3^-]/[CO_2]$ ratio
b. The net result of a metabolic acidosis is a decreased HCO_3^- concentration
c. A metabolic acidosis may be compensated for by hyperventilating
d. Respiratory acidosis is secondary to impaired alveolar ventilation
e. Acute respiratory acidosis is compensated for by increased renal bicarbonate production

An acidosis of whatever origin may be defined as a decrease in the $[HCO_3^-]/[CO_2]$ ratio. In a metabolic acidosis there is a net decrease in bicarbonate concentration. This may be caused by decreased bicarbonate production, excess loss of bicarbonate, or by an increase in acid production which binds the bicarbonate to produce H_2CO_3. A metabolic acidosis is compensated for by hyperventilating, which reduces the carbon dioxide concentration and so restores the $[HCO_3^-]/[CO_2]$ ratio. Respiratory acidosis may be acute or chronic but both result from impaired alveolar ventilation. The former cannot be compensated for to any significant degree by renal mechanisms.

323

4.8 *Causes of alkalosis*

a. Alkalosis is caused by a rise in the ratio $[HCO_3^-]/[CO_2]$
b. A respiratory alkalosis is commonly seen in obstructive airways disease
c. A metabolic alkalosis may be caused by pyloric stenosis
d. A metabolic alkalosis is well compensated for by respiratory mechanisms
e. A respiratory alkalosis may be caused by an increased intracranial pressure

An alkalosis of whatever origin may be defined as an increase in the $[HCO_3^-]/[CO_2]$ ratio. During vomiting there will be loss of acidic gastric contents and of alkaline duodenal juices and therefore a metabolic alkalosis does not always occur. However, there is no compensatory loss of alkaline duodenal juices in

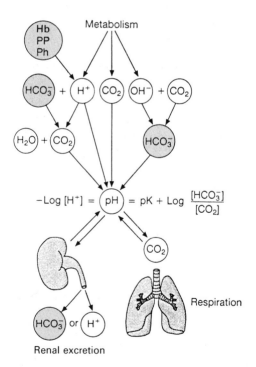

Fig 119 **Regulation of the blood pH.** ⊚ **Buffering agent: Hb, haemoglobin; PP, plasma proteins; Ph. phosphate**

pyloric stenosis and vomiting invariably results in a metabolic alkalosis. Hyperventilation can never compensate for a metabolic alkalosis because CO_2 retention will eventually stimulate the respiratory centres and increase ventilation. Chronic bronchitics are usually in a state of respiratory acidosis secondary to retention of CO_2. A raised intracranial pressure can cause hyperventilation and a resultant respiratory alkalosis.

5: Muscle physiology

5.1 Properties of striated muscle

a. Fibres are arranged in a fusiform manner
b. Striated muscle has a transverse tubular system which acts as a calcium reserve
c. The longitudinal tubular system is a continuation of the sarcolemma
d. Fast twitch fibres are more fatigueable than slow twitch fibres
e. Slow twitch fibres have a higher myoglobin concentration than fast twitch fibres

Striated muscle fibrils are organised into units known as sarcomeres. Postsynaptic potentials spread through the muscle via the transverse tubular system, which is an extension of the sarcolemma. The longitudal tubular system runs parallel to the myofibrils and functions as the calcium reservoir; it is a continuation of the sarcoplasmic reticulum. Fast twitch fibres are designed for anaerobic activity and are more fatigueable than slow twitch fibres, which are rich in myoglobin.

5.2 The sarcomere

a. The sarcomere is the portion of the myofibril between two Z lines
b. Actin and myosin fibrils overlap in the A band
c. The H band consists solely of actin
d. The length of the sarcomere is 1.5–3.2 μm
e. Sarcomeres are found in skeletal and cardiac muscle

325

The sarcomere is the functional unit of striated muscle fibrils and is the region between two Z lines. The A band is the region where the myosin and actin fibres overlap. The H band is found in the middle of the A band and consists only of myosin. The sarcomere varies in length from 1.5 to 3.2 μm, the optimum length being 3–3.2 μm. This is the region of maximal tension on the length/tension curve. Both striated and cardiac muscle are organised in sarcomeres.

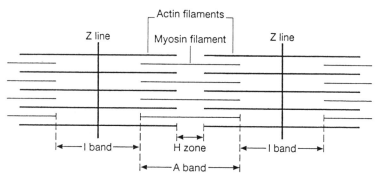

Fig 120 The sarcomere

5.3 *Events in skeletal muscle contraction*

a. An action potential causes a calcium influx from the extracellular space
b. Calcium binds to tropinin
c. Actin–myosin cross bridges form
d. GDP bound to the myosin head is split by the GTPase in actin
e. Magnesium is essential for contraction

An action potential travelling in the transverse tubular system causes calcium release from the longitudinal tubular system. The calcium binds to tropinin subunits (found on tropomyosin which is wound around the actin filament) and frees the myosin binding sites, which then combine with actin to form "cross bridges". The myosin ATPase splits an ATP molecule with the aid of magnesium, and the resultant energy is used to hinge the ratchet mechanism of the myosin heads.

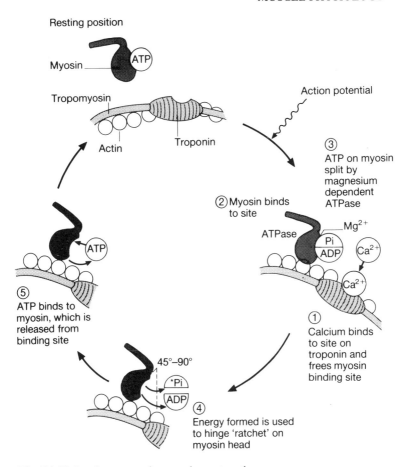

Fig 121 Molecular events in muscle contraction

5.4 *Features of motor endplates*

a. Motor endplates are found in all types of muscle
b. Acetylcholine is the neurotransmitter
c. Acetylcholine release is initiated by an efflux of calcium from the nerve endings
d. Curare blocks transmission
e. The action of acetylcholine is rapidly reduced by reuptake into the nerve terminal

Motor endplates are found only in skeletal muscle. Acetylcholine, which is found in vesicles, is released into the synaptic cleft when an action potential causes a calcium influx into the neurone. Curare displaces acetylcholine from its postsynaptic binding site but does not itself produce a depolarisation. The action of acetylcholine is terminated by the choline esterase enzyme, unlike that of noradrenaline which relies on reuptake across the presynaptic membrane.

5.5 *Electrical activity in skeletal muscle*

a. A change in the endplate potential is produced by sodium influx
b. The action potential produced is approximately 2–5 ms long
c. The frequency of action potentials needed to produce tetanus in fast twitch fibres is 60–100 Hz
d. Skeletal muscle has a longer refractory period than cardiac muscle
e. Succinylcholine will produce a postsynaptic potential

When acetylcholine binds to its postsynaptic receptor it triggers an influx of sodium ions, which produce an excitatory postsynaptic potential. Temporal or spatial summation of these potentials may enable thresholds to be reached and a postsynaptic action potential produced. This action potential is 2–5 ms long but frequencies of up to 100 Hz will not produce tetany in fast twitch muscles. The long refractory period of cardiac muscle means that tetanus can not be produced. Succinylcholine will cause initial depolarisation of the postsynaptic membrane before causing neuromuscular blockage.

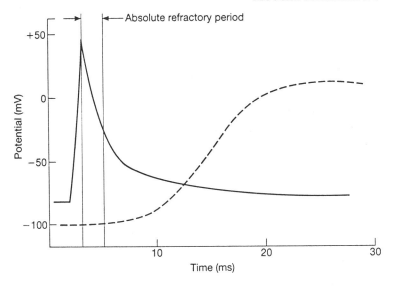

Fig 122 The striated muscle action potential. — Action potential; ---
mechanical tension

5.6 *Properties of cardiac, smooth, and skeletal muscle*

> a. The action potential of cardiac muscle has a plateau and is
>   approximately 200 ms
> b. The heart has no motor units
> c. Skeletal muscle normally operates on the plateau of the
>   length/tension curve
> d. Both visceral smooth muscle and cardiac muscle have a
>   pacemaker function
> e. A smooth muscle contraction follows approximately
>   150 ms after the action potential

The cardiac muscle action potential has a characteristic plateau
caused by the slow influx of calcium ions, and has a duration of
approximately 200 ms. Skeletal muscle, unlike cardiac muscle,
operates at the peak of the length/tension curve and is the only
type of muscle that does not require an intrinsic pacemaker.
The smooth muscle contraction is a slow rising one that begins
approximately 150 ms after the action potential.

329

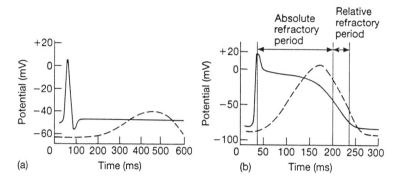

Fig 123 Action potential (—) and mechanical tension (---) of (a) smooth muscle; (b) cardiac muscle

5.7 The muscle spindle

a. Intrafusal fibres are of two types
b. Ia afferents have annulospiral endings
c. γ Efferents stimulate extrafusal fibres
d. Muscle spindles respond primarily to a change in muscle tension
e. The stretch reflex is monosynaptic

The muscle spindle is the main regulatory unit of skeletal muscle. Its intrafusal fibres are of two types: nuclear bag and nuclear chain fibres. The Ia afferents arising from the annulospiral endings on these fibres travel to the spinal cord where they make a monosynaptic connection with α motor neurones. These supply extrafusal fibres of the same muscle. The endings of the γ efferent fibres terminate either on nuclear bag fibres as plate endings, or on nuclear chain fibres as trail endings. Stimulation of the γ efferent system shortens the intrafusal fibres so initiating impulses in the Ia fibres. This can lead to reflex contraction of the muscle. Increased γ efferent discharge thus increases spindle sensitivity, and the sensitivity of the spindles to stretch varies with the rate of γ efferent discharge. The spindle responds primarily to changes in muscle length, not to changes in muscle tension, which is the function of the golgi tendon organ.

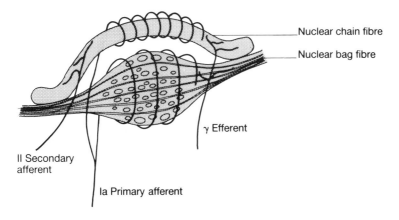

Nuclear chain fibre

Nuclear bag fibre

γ Efferent

II Secondary
afferent

Ia Primary afferent

Fig 124 The muscle spindle

6: The central nervous system

6.1 *Mechanisms involved in establishing the resting membrane potential*

a. Active transport of sodium into and potassium out of the cell
b. A cell membrane with a low sodium conductance
c. A cell membrane that is permeable to proteins and phosphates
d. A potassium conductance greater than a sodium conductance
e. A very low chloride conductance

The resting potential of the cell is due to the uneven distribution of cations and anions between the intracellular and extracellular fluid according to an electrochemical gradient. Cell membranes have a low sodium conductance and sodium is actively pumped out of the cell against a chemical gradient. Potassium conductance is relatively high so potassium has a tendency to leak out of cells. This is counteracted by its active transport in the opposite direction. Chloride conductance, unlike that of other anions (such as proteins and phosphates), is relatively high. The negative resting potential tends to drive chloride out of the cell against its chemical gradient.

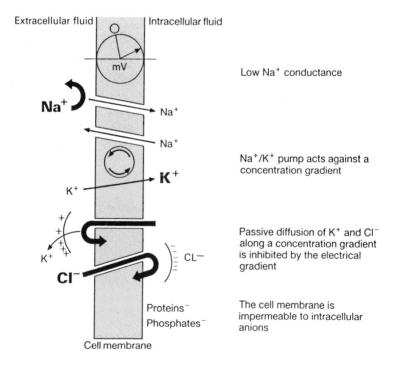

Extracellular fluid   Intracellular fluid

mV

Na⁺

Na⁺

Na⁺

K⁺

K⁺

K⁺

Cl⁻

CL⁻

Proteins⁻

Phosphates⁻

Cell membrane

Low Na⁺ conductance

Na⁺/K⁺ pump acts against a concentration gradient

Passive diffusion of K⁺ and Cl⁻ along a concentration gradient is inhibited by the electrical gradient

The cell membrane is impermeable to intracellular anions

Fig 125 Formation of the resting potential

6.2 *Properties of the action potential*

a. An action potential is generated only when stimulation is sufficient to produce a change in potential great enough to reach the threshold potential
b. Depolarisation is caused by an influx of sodium ions
c. Sodium conductance increases uniformly throughout the action potential
d. The membrane potential reaches positive values
e. Repolarisation is caused by a slow rise in potassium conductance

The initial depolarisation is caused by a slow increase in the sodium conductance. However, an action potential will be produced only if the threshold is reached and sodium channels are activated, resulting in a massive influx of sodium ions. During this depolarisation phase, the membrane potential will reach positive values. Repolarisation is secondary to a decrease in the sodium conductance and a slow increase in the potassium conductance, which allows potassium to diffuse out of the cell. The membrane potential difference may become greater than the original resting potential—this is called hyperpolarisation.

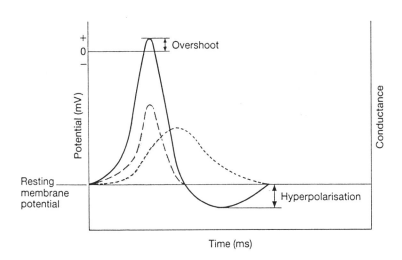

Fig 126 Sodium (—) and potassium (----) conductances during the action potential

6.3 *Types of nerve fibres*

> a. Aα Fibres are found in muscle spindle afferents and skeletal muscle efferents
> b. Aγ Fibres are muscle spindle efferents
> c. C Fibres are fast pain fibres
> d. Aα Fibres have a conduction of velocity of 70–120 m/s
> e. B Fibres are unmyelinated

Aα Fibres have the largest diameter of any nerve fibre and have a conduction velocity of 70–120 m/s. They are found in the muscle spindle afferents and skeletal muscle efferents. Aγ Fibres innervate the intrafusal fibres of muscle spindles. C Fibres are the only unmyelinated fibres. They are responsible for "slow" pain conduction, and postganglionic autonomic conduction. Aδ Fibres are responsible for "fast" pain conduction.

Answers

1.1	a, b, c	**3.3**	b, c, d, e	**4.7**	a, b, d
1.2	c, d, e	**3.4**	b, c, e	**4.8**	a, c, e
1.3	b, c, d	**3.5**	a, b, c, d, e		
1.4	a, c, d, e	**3.6**	c, d	**5.1**	d, e
1.5	a, b, c, e	**3.7**	b, c, e	**5.2**	a, b, d, e
1.6	a, c, d, e	**3.8**	b, c, e	**5.3**	b, c, e
1.7	a, b, e	**3.9**	b, c, d, e	**5.4**	b, d
1.8	a, b, c, e	**3.10**	a, b, c	**5.5**	a, b, e
		3.11	a, c, d, e	**5.6**	a, b, c, d, e
2.1	a, b, e			**5.7**	a, b, e
2.2	b, c, d	**4.1**	a, b, c, e		
2.3	a, b, d	**4.2**	b, c, e	**6.1**	b, c, d
2.4	a, b, d	**4.3**	c, e	**6.2**	a, b, d, e
		4.4	a, c	**6.3**	a, b, d
3.1	b, d, e	**4.5**	a, b, d, e		
3.2	c, e	**4.6**	a, b, c, e		

Index

abducent nerve 3, 51, 55, 68
acanthamoeba 124–5
accessory nerve 74
accommodation 180–1, 216,
    220–1, 223–4
acetazolamide 188–9
acetylcholine 180, 182, 201, 233,
    234, 261, 328
acetylcholinesterase 234
acid-base balance 318
acidosis 323
acinar cells 7
acoustic neuromas 55
actin 326
Actinomyces israeli 99
action potential 333
acute inflammation 135
    cellular phase 136
    complement system 141
    natural history 142
    plasma cascade systems 142–3
    vascular phase 135–6
acyclovir 131
adaptation *see* visual adaptation
adenosine triphosphatase 326
    see also sodium potassium
        ATPase
adenosine triphosphate
    (ATP) 219, 250
adenoviruses 111
adenylate cyclase 210, 255
Adie's pupil 61, 181, 238
Adie's syndrome 223
adrenal cortex 313
adrenal medulla 315
adrenaline 186, 206, 236, 302,
    315, 316
adrenergic system 184–6
adrenocorticotrophic
    hormone 313
AIDS 109, 117, 118, 133
albinos 282
albumin 199, 211, 310, 313

alcohol 232
aldosterone 302, 320, 322
alkalosis 324–5
allergic reaction 154
amacrine cells 37
amblyopia 276
amino acids 217, 251, 311, 312,
    320
γ-aminobutyric acid 261
amiodarone 194, 195
amphetamine 232
amphotericin 128–9
anaemia 129, 307, 318
    aplastic 128
anaerobic ocular pathogens 99
anaesthetics, ocular 192
anaphylatoxins 141
aneurysms 53, 167, 168, 231
angiotensin II 302, 322
angular vein 9
anisocoria 228, 236
Annulus of Zinn 49
ansa cervicalis 75–6
anterior ethmoidal nerve 56
antibiotics 129–30
antidiuretic hormone 317, 320,
    322
antifungal agents 128–9
antigens 149, 156, 161
antimicrobial agents 125–9
antimitotic chemotherapy 193
aorta 299, 301, 304
aqueous
    blood barrier 208–9
    composition 211
    dynamics 212
    functions 210
    outflow mechanics 212
    protein content 211
    refractive index 17
arachidonic acid 138
Arden ratio 266
Argyll Robertson pupil 237

arterioles 41, 299
Arthus reaction 157, 158
ascorbic acid 211
L-aspartate 261
Aspergillus fumigatus 120
asteroid hyalosis 225
asthma 185, 308
astrocytes 43
atherosclerosis
  natural history 168
  plaques 166–7
  risk factors 169
atlas 74
atropine 179, 183, 232
auricular nerves 76
autocrine growth factors 172–3
autoimmune disease 157
autonomic nervous system 58–63
axis 74
azathioprine 193

β blockers 185, 311
B cells 146, 148, 159–60, 190
bacille-Calmette-Guérin 94
bacilli 93–9
  gram negative 98, 126, 127
  gram positive 96, 125
Bacillus anthracis 95
Bacillus brevis 95
Bacillus cereus 95, 96
bacteria
  culture 88
  gram staining 88
  killing 139
  metabolism and growth 87
  pathogenicity 89
  sporing 94
  structure 86
  toxins 89
Bacteroides 126, 127
Bainbridge reflex 304
baroreceptors 304
Behçet's disease 193
Bell's phenomenon 201
benoxinate 192
betaxolol 185
bicarbonate 188, 318, 323
biliary leaks 323
binocular vision 276, 292–4
bipolar cells 37

blepharitis 98, 99
blepharospasm 201
blindness
  cortical 47
  night 263
blinking
  reflex 12, 199
  spontaneous 200
blood aqueous barrier 208–9
blood flow
  autoregulation 299–300
  axial streaming 136
  hormonal control 302
  neuronal control 301
  physics 300
  transcapillary exchange 302
blood pH 324
blood pressure 303–4, 316, 319
blood transfusion 156
blood vessels 299
blood volume 299
blue cones 282, 283
body water 320, 321
botulinum toxin 201
Bowman's membrane 18, 203
brachiocephalic artery 76
bradycardia 304
bradykinin 142, 302
brain abscess 118
brain stem 6, 54, 59
bregma 69
Broca-Sulza effect 285
Brodman's area 17 *see* visual
  cortex
bronchitis 325
bronchospasm 185, 316
Brucella abortus 98
brucellosis 127
Brubaker's correction 213
Bruch's membrane 32–3
burns 98, 323

calcarine sulcus 46, 47, 275
calcium 138, 163, 325, 326, 329
caloric testing 247
Candida albicans 119
capillaries 299, 301, 302–3
  glomerular 319
  retinal 41
capsids 101

carbachol 180, 234
carbon dioxide 87, 305, 323, 325
  alveolar partial pressure 309
carbon monoxide 306
carbonic anhydrase 188, 210
  inhibitors 189
carcinogens 175
carcinoma *in situ* 171
cardiac failure 304
cardiac muscle 326, 329
cardiac output 304, 316
cardiovascular pathology 162
cardiovascular
    physiology 299–305
carotid arteries 44, 64, 68, 76–8,
    81
  sheath 77
  sinus 76, 304
cataractogenesis 220
cataracts 110, 182, 190, 191, 195,
    218, 230
  diabetic 219
catecholamines 314
  half life 316
  properties 184, 315–16
  receptors 184
cavernous sinus 64, 67–8
  thrombosis 15, 55, 66, 68
CD cells 115, 149
ceftazidime 126
cefuroxime 126
cell cycle 170
cell death 103
cell mediated
    hypersensitivity 158, 159
cell mediated immunity 150
cell membranes 331
central nervous system 331–4
central retinal artery 41, 43, 64,
    256
  occlusion 122, 265
cephalosporins 126, 130
cerebellopontine angle
    tumours 200
cerebellum 243
cerebral arteries 44, 48
cervical plexus 75–6
cervical proprioceptors 243
cervical vertebrae 74
cestode infections 122

chalones 172
chemical carcinogens 175
chemotaxis 137–8
chickenpox 108
Chlamydia trachomatis 100–1
chloramphenicol 127–8, 194
chloride 199, 204, 217, 332
chloroquine 194
cholesterol 313
cholineacetyl transferase 180
cholinergic agonists 180–3, 232,
    233
cholinesterase 180, 328
chorda tympani 74, 82
chorioretinitis 109, 118
choroid 31-2
  circulation 265
  disease 265
  embryology 31
ciliary arteries 15, 27, 32, 64,
    65–6
ciliary body
  blood supply 26
  embryology 22
  epithelium 23
  structure 22
ciliary epithelium 207
ciliary ganglion 61, 231, 234, 238
ciliary muscle 23
  innervation 27, 28
  properties 223
ciliary nerves 15, 19, 28, 32, 231
cilioretinal artery 41
Circle of Zinn 45, 65
clostridia 95–6
Clostridium perfringens 96, 99
Clostridium tetani 96
clotting 142
coagulase 89
cocaine 186, 192, 201, 232, 236
cocci 91–3, 127
codeine 155
collagen 226–7
  lattice 205–6
collarette 25
coloboma 24, 42
Colorado tick virus 104
colour vision 290–2
coma 323
commensals 91

complement fixation test 104, 105
cones 37, 38, 40, 259, 260
  colour vision 290
  sensitivity 289
congenital abnormalities 110
conjunctiva 10
  blood supply 14
  histology 15
  innervation 14
  structure 14
conjunctival veins 15
conjunctivitis 98, 99, 109
  acute haemorrhagic 112
  bacterial 100, 128
contact dermatitis 158
contact lenses 125
contrast sensitivity 285–6
Corie cycle 251
cornea
  angle anatomy 21
  avascular 206
  biochemistry 203
  dehydration 205
  deposits 194
  development 16
  electrolyte and glucose
    content 204
  embryology 16
  endothelium/epithelium 19
  innervation 19
  limbus 20
  nerves 16
  pharmacokinetics 178
  physical properties 202
  sensation 207
  structure 17, 203
  transparency 205
  trauma 98
  ulcers 98
  wounds 206
corneoscleral junction 20
corticosteroids 179, 194, 195
  anti-inflammatory actions 189
  effects 190, 313–14
  production 313
  raised intraocular pressure 191
  side effects 190–1
  systemic 190
corticotrophin releasing
  hormone 314

Corynebacterium diphtheriae 96
cottonwool spots 118
Coxsackie viruses 112
cranial nerves 52–8
Cryptococcus neoformans 119
crystallins 218
curare 328
Cushing's syndrome 314
cyclic AMP 138, 163, 209–10, 313
cyclic GMP 138, 255
cyclopentolate 183, 232
cycloplegia 183
cyclosporin 193
cysticercosis 122
cytokines 150
cytomegalovirus 103, 108–9
  retinitis 109, 118, 132, 133

dacryoadenitis 111
dacryocystorrhinostomy 9
dark adaptation 229, 262, 263,
  266, 286, 287, 288, 289
deafness 110
De Lange's contrast
  sensitivity 286
Demodex foliicularum 91
Descemet's membrane 16, 18, 203
dexamethasone 191
diabetes 169, 188, 311
  cataract formation 219
  ketoacidosis 312
  retinopathy 191
diaphragm 76
dichromats 291
diencephalon 35
dihydroxyacetone phosphate 251
dilator pupillae 25, 27
diplopia 294–5
disinfection 90
DNA 251
DNA viruses 102
Donder's law 241
dopamine 184
dorsal motor nucleus 59
dorsal nasal artery 64
Down's syndrome 175
drug transport, intraocular 178
dysplasia 171

echinococcus granulosus 122
echothiopate 182
echoviruses 112
ectropion uvae 26
Edinger-Westphal nucleus 28, 59, 63, 232
edrophonium 201
electro-oculogram 266–7
electrodiagnostic tests 261–71
electroretinograms 261–5
emboli 165–6
encephalitis 109
endocrinology 309–13
endophthalmitis 97, 99
endothelin 300
endotoxins 90
entamoeba 128
enterobacteriaceae 97
enteroviruses 111–12
eosinophils 152, 153
episclera 34
Epstein-Barr virus 104, 176, 177
ergosterol 129
erythropoietin 318
Escherichia coli 97, 99, 125
ethambutol 194
ethmoidal arteries 64
ethmoidal sinus 4, 5
excyclotorsion 240, 241, 242
exotoxins 90
extracellular isotonic volume depletion 321
extraocular muscles 48–52, 239–247
  control 242, 243
  innervation 51
  palsies 111
  relations 51–2
eyelids 9–13
  associated eye movements 200
  blinking 12, 199–200
  blood supply 13
  drug effects 201
  innervation 13
  lymphatic drainage 13
  structure 10

facial artery 13, 80
facial muscles 83
facial nerve 71, 81

Ferry-Porter Law 286
fibrillary twitching 201
fibrinolytic systems 142
fibrinopeptides 142
fibroblasts 25, 31, 144, 314
fibronectin 173
Fick's axes 239
fixation movements 245
flicker electroretinogram 263, 264
flickering light source 284–5, 286
flora 91
Floren's Law 246
flucloxacillin 125
fluconazole 125
flucytosine 129, 130
fluoromethalone 179
foramina 73–4
forced expiratory volume 308
forced vital capacity 308
foscarnet 133
fovea centralis 38, 40, 280, 281–3
foveola 40
Francisella tularensis 98
Frisby test 297
frontal bone 1
frontal nerve 3, 52, 56
frontal sinus 4, 5
fructose 6-phosphate 249
fungi 118–120

galactilol 220
gamma radiation 90
ganciclovir 131–2
ganglion cells 37, 40, 43, 265, 272
  midget 280, 282
gas gangrene 96
gaze palsy, vertical 231
gaze positions 239
genetic disorders 175
genital infection 106, 119
Gennari's stripe 273
gentamicin 126–7
giardia 128
gingivostomatitis 106
glands of Moll 10
glands of Zeis 10
glaucoma 110, 181, 182, 183, 191
glial cells 39
glossopharyngeal nerves 304
glucagon 249, 251, 311, 312–13

gluconeogenesis 251, 312, 313
glucose 199, 204, 211, 217, 219, 225, 311, 314, 320
glucose 6-phosphatase 248
glutathione 219, 220
glycerin 205
glycerol 187–8, 251
glycine 261
glycogen 312
glycolysis 219, 248–9
glycoproteins 225
  HIV 117
glycosaminoglycans 203, 204
goblet cells 15
gonococcus 93
Gradenigo's syndrome 55
graft rejection 156, 161–2
graft versus host reactions 190
Gram staining 88–9
granuloma 144–5
Graves' disease 193
guanethedine 186, 201

haematoma, extradural 69, 231
haemoglobin 305–6
haemolysins 89
Haemophilus influenzae 125, 128
haemorrhage 323
Hageman factor 142
head
  anatomy 74–84
  tilt 54
headache 181, 194
Heaf test 159
heart disease 110, 185
helminths 120–1, 122
  immunity to 152–4
hemianopias 46
hepatitis B 103,104,112,115–17,176
  serology 113
Hering's law 244
heroin 232
herpes gladiatorum 106
herpes simplex virus 103, 104
  infections 118, 131, 133
  latency 107
  pathogenicity 106
  subtypes 106
herpes viruses 105–9
herpes zoster 56, 118

herpes zoster ophthalmicus 193
heterophorias 295
heterotropias 294, 295
hexokinase 249
hexose-monophosphate shunt 219
hiatus semilunaris 4
hippus 228
histamine 136, 155, 302
histoplasmosis 118
HIV 114–18
  immune response 115
  life cycle 116
  ocular manifestations 117–18
  pathogenesis 114–15
  serology 117
HLA 149, 160–1
homatropine 183, 232
horizontal cells 37
Horner's syndrome 186, 201, 234, 236
human immunodeficiency virus *see* HIV
human papillomavirus 176
Hurler's syndrome 199
Hutchinson's sign 56
hyaloid artery 35
hyaluronic acid 225
hyaluronidase 89
hydatid disease 122
hydrogen peroxide 139, 219
hydroxyamphetamine 186, 234, 236
hyperlipidaemia 169
hyperosmotic agents 187
hyperplasia 171
hyperpolarisation 333
hypersensitivity reactions 120
  Type I 154–5
  Type II 156
  Type III 157
  Type IV 158–9
hypertension 169
  ocular 268
hypertrophy 171
hyperventilation 323, 325
hypoglycaemia 315
hypoglycaemics, oral 194
hypoglossal canal 74
hypoglossal nerve 75
hypoproteinaemia 302

hypothalamic-pituitary system 317, 318
hypotonic fluid loss 323

immune complexes 157
immunocompromised patient 98, 109, 119. 120
immunoglobulin A 199
immunoglobulin G 199, 211
immunoglobulins 146–8
incyclotorsion 240, 241, 242
inferior colliculus 243
inferior orbital fissure 2, 3
inferior salivatory nucleus 59
inflammation 135–45
    chronic 144–5
    natural history 142
infraorbital nerve 6, 13, 57
infratemporal fossa 84
infratrochlear nerve 13
inotropic drugs 304
insulin 311–12
interferons 150, 151, 152
interleukins 150, 151
interstitial fluid 318, 321
intracranial pressure 45, 194, 231, 325
intraocular pressure 205, 231, 256
    diurnal variation 214
    drug effects 181, 182, 183, 184, 185, 186, 187
    mean value 215
    population distribution 215
    steroids 191
iodine 309
irin 209
iris 182, 208–9
    blood supply 26
    damage 231
    embryology 24
    epthelial development 24
    epithelium 26
    innervation 27, 28
    muscle 24
    structure 25
iron 98, 307
islets of Langerhans 311, 312
isotonic fluid loss 323

jugular foramen 74

jugular veins 78
Jones-Mote reaction 158

keratitis 118, 125, 185, 191
    necrotising 99
    nummular 98
keratoconjunctivitis 111
ketoconazole 125, 129
kidney see renal
kinins 136, 142, 318
Klebsiella 97
Klinefelter's syndrome 175
Koch-Weeks bacillus 98
Krause glands 15, 197
Krebs' cycle 203, 250

lacrimal canaliculi 7, 99
lacrimal ducts 5
lacrimal gland 196
    drainage 7
    histology 7
    parasympathetic innervation 6
    structure 5
lacrimal nerve 3, 6, 52, 56
lacrimal sac 8–9
lactate 211, 248, 249
lambda 69
lamina cribrosa 34
lamina fusca 34
lamina papyrecia 2
La Place's law 301
laryngeal nerves 78
lateral geniculate nuclei 46, 48, 272–3
lateral palpebral raphe 10
lens
    biochemistry 217
    capsule 222
    embryology 29
    functions 216
    histology 30
    metabolism 218–19
    optics 216
    placode 29
    proteins 217–18
    structure 29
levator palpebrae superioris 11, 12
light adaptation 266, 286
lipids 219

lipolysis 312
lipoproteins 169
Listeria monocytogenes 96
liver 122
    damage 129
lung 300
    perfusion 308–9
    tumour 236
    volume 307–8
lymph nodes 5, 13, 146
lymphatic drainage 5, 13, 79, 302
lymphocytes 104, 108
    see also B cells, T cells
lymphogranuloma venereum 100
lymphokines 146, 150, 151
lysine oxidation 227
lysosomes 258
    enzymes 310
    membranes 189
lysozyme 199

MacConkey Agar 88
macrophages 115, 136, 139–40,
    144
macula lutea 39–40, 47
macular disease 109, 271
macular dystrophy 267
"macular sparing" 48
magnesium 326
major histocompatibility
    complex 149
mandibular nerve 84
mannitol 187
Marcus Gunn syndrome 201
Marfan's syndrome 227
mast cells 154-5
maxilla 1, 71–2
maxillary artery 77, 84
maxillary nerve 3, 57
maxillary sinus 4, 5, 72
Mazzotti skin test 121
measles 109
medial palpebral ligament 9, 10
Meibomian glands 10
melanin 257, 283
melanocytes 25, 31
melanosomes 258
melatonin 259
meningeal arteries 69, 73
meninges 42, 43

meningitis 106, 128
meningococcus 93
meningoencephalitis 111, 119
mercaptopurine 193
mesangial cells 319
mesosomes 86
metaplasia 171
metarhodopsins 255
metastasis 174
methaemoglobin 307
methylene blue 89
metronidazole 128
microphthalmia 109, 110
mid brain 28, 53
    lesions 231
middle cranial fossa 2
    foramina 73
mineralocorticoids 313
miosis 180, 234, 235
mitochondria 248, 250
monochromats 282, 291
monocytes 104, 115
monokines 150
Moraxella lacunata 98
morphine 155
motor endplates 327
moulds 118
mucopolysaccharides 203
Müller cells 37, 39, 248, 258
Müller's muscle 12, 186
mumps 111
muramic acid 86
muscarinic agonists 180–2
muscarinic antagonists 182–3
muscles
    cardiac 329
    contraction 326–7
    skeletal 328–9
    smooth 329
    spindle 330
    striated 325
mycobacteria 93–4
mydriasis 181, 182, 184, 186, 190,
    232, 233
mydriatic agents 232
myoepithelial cells 7
myofibroblasts 144
myoglobin 306, 325
myopia 191
myosin 326

NADPH 251
nasal septum 56, 62
nasociliary nerve 3, 52, 56
nasolacrimal duct 2, 8–9, 72
nasopharynx 62, 93
near triad 221
neck 74–84
Neisseriae 93
nematodes 121, 153
neomycin 125
neoplasia
  characteristics 170
  formation 172
  invasion 173
  malignant 172
nerve fibres 334
nervus intermedius 6, 82
neuroglial cells 39, 43
neurotransmitters 261
neutropenia 132
neutrophils 136
newborn 283
nicotine 232
night blindness 263
nitric oxide 300
Nocardia asteroides 96
noradrenaline 201, 232, 233, 234,
    261, 302
  conversion 315
  effects 316
nose 56, 62, 72
nucleic acids 102
nystagmus 195, 282, 283
  optokinetic 244, 245–6

oblique muscles 50, 240
ocular anatomy 10
ocular movements 239–247
  smooth pursuit 244
ocular trauma 97
oculomotor nerve 3, 12, 51, 52–3
  lesions 231, 237
oedema 302
Oncherca volvulus 121
onchocerciasis 121
oncogenes 174, 176–7
ophthalmia 193
ophthalmia neonatorum 93
ophthalmic artery 3, 45, 64
ophthalmic nerve 52, 56

ophthalmic veins 3, 66
opioid peptides 315
opsonisation 139, 148
optic canal 3, 43
optic chiasma 44
  compression 271
  lesions 46
optic cup 35
optic disc 43
optic nerve 42–3
  blood supply 45
  demyelination 270
  disease 230, 268, 271, 292
  relations 43
optic tracts 48
optic vesicle 35–6
optokinetic nystagmus 244, 245–6
optotypes 277
ora serrata 36
orbicularis oculi 12–13
orbit 1–2
  blood vessels 64–6
  fissures 2
  septum 9
orchitis 111
ouabain 205
oxidation 87
oxygen 203, 248, 249, 250
  alveolar partial pressure 308
  binding protein 306–7
  consumption 311
  dissociation of
    haemoglobin 305–6

pain 5, 207, 334
palate 62, 72
palatine bone 1
palisades of Vogt 20
palpebral arteries 13, 15
palpebral fissure 10
palpebral ligaments 10
Pancoast tumour 236
pancreatitis 111
Panum's area 292, 293, 294
papilloedema 45, 194
paramyxoviruses 103
paranasal sinuses 3–4
parasympathetic nerves 28
  nuclei 59–60
Parinaud's syndrome 231

parotid gland 59, 77, 80
Pasteurella multocida 98
pasteurisation 90
pattern electroretinogram 265, 267–8
penicillins 125
pentose phosphate pathway 251–2
perinatal period 275–6
petrosal nerves 6, 73, 82
phagocytosis 138–9
pharmacokinetics 178–9
pharyngoconjunctival fever 111
phenylephrine 182, 186, 232
phenylethanolamine-*N*-methyl-transferase 315
phenytoin 195
phosphate preparations 179
phospholipase A 138
photophobia 282
photopic electroretinogram 263, 264
photoreceptors 36, 37, 38, 40, 259–60, 286, 288
phrenic nerve 76
physostigmine 182, 234
pial arteries 48
pilocarpine 179, 180, 181, 182
pituitary fossa 68
pituitary hormones 317
Pityrosporon orbiculari 91
plasma cascade systems 142, 143
plasma osmolarity 320, 321
plasminogen 211
plasmids 86
platelet factor 3 162
platelets 162–3
platyhelminths 121
Poiseuille Hagen Formula 212, 301
polioviruses 112
posterior communicating artery aneurysm 53, 231
potassium 199, 204, 211, 217, 225, 320, 331, 333
   see also sodium potassium ATPase
pregnancy 108, 110, 123, 127, 128
proparacaine 192
Propionibacterium acne 91, 99
prostaglandins 136, 163, 209, 318

protanopes 290–1
proteins 251, 310, 314
   lens 217–8
   oxygen binding 306–7
proteus 97, 127
protonomalous person 290–1
protozoa 120–5, 152–4
Pseudomonas aeruginosa 98, 126, 127
pseudotumour cerebrae 194
pterion 69
pterygoid canal 6
pterygoid venous plexus 66
pterygopalatine fossa 2, 6
pterygopalatine ganglion 57, 62–3
ptosis 190, 201
pulvinar 274
pupil
   defects 230
   effects of increasing size 229
   light near dissociation 237
   light reflexes 230
   normal 228
   pathways 62
   reactions to light 228
pyloric stenosis 325
pyramidal cells 273
pyruvate 249

Q fever 127

rabies 103
rectus muscles 12, 48–9, 240
   palsy 296
red blood cells 104
renal impairment 187, 189, 193
renal physiology
   extracellular isotonic volume depletion 321
   functions of kidney 317
   glomerular filtration 319
   glomerulotubular balance 320
   plasma osmolality 320, 321
   tubules 319–320
respiration 307–8
respiratory acidosis 323
respiratory physiology 305–9
resting membrane potential 331
retina 248–260, 311
   blood supply 40–1, 255–6

cells 39
cottonwool spots 118
differentiation 36
disease 267
embryology 35–6
haemorrhage 122
membranes 39
metabolism 248
necrosis 99
neural 36–7
photochemistry 255
photoreceptors 36, 37, 38, 259–60
pigment epithelium 258
T. gondii infection 124
retinal 253
retinal arteries 41
retinal veins 256
retinitis 119
CMV 109, 118, 132, 133
retinoblastoma 175, 177
retinol *see* vitamin A
retinoschisis 263
retinosis pigmentosa 263
retromandibular vein 81
rhesus incompatibility 156
rheumatoid arthritis 157, 193
rhodopsin 255, 288
rifampicin 130
RNA 127, 251
RNA viruses 102
rods 37, 38, 259, 260, 286
sensitivity 288
rubella 103, 109–10

saccadic movements 244
saccule 243
salivary glands 301
salmonella 97
sarcomeres 325–6
schistosomiasis 122
Schlemm's canal 21, 212, 213
Schwalbe's line 20, 21
sclera 33–4
embryology 31
histology 34
melting 191
scleritis 193
scotopic electroretinogram 263, 264

scotopic system 286
semicircular canals 243, 246
sharks 205
shingles 107
sialic acid 225
silver nitrate 93
sinus infection 5
skull
bones 70–2
fissures 73–4
foramina 73
fractures 1, 57, 69, 231
sutures 69
smallpox 104
smoking 169
Snellen letters 277
sodium 188, 211, 225, 255, 321, 322, 328
conductance 331, 333
sodium potassium ATPase 204, 205, 209, 217, 219, 220
insulin 312
sorbitol 219
spatial contrast sensitivity function 277–9
spectral sensitivity 283
sphenoid bone 1, 70
sphenoidal sinuses 4, 5
spincter pupillae 25, 27
Spiral of Tilau 49
squint *See* strabismus
standard luminosity function 291
staphylococci 91–2, 125, 126
Staphylococcus aureus 91, 92, 125
Staphylococcus epidermis 91, 92
Starling hypothesis 302
Starling's law 304–5
stellate cells 273
stereopsis 274, 292, 296–7
sterilisation 90
sternocleidomastoid 75
Stiles-Crawford effect 229
strabismus 49, 109, 181, 295
streptococci 92, 125
Streptococcus pneumoniae 93
Streptococcus pyogenes 93
stress 312
striate cortex *see* visual cortex
stroke volume 304
stylomastoid foramen 71, 74

subacute sclerosing
    panencephalitis 109
submandibular gland 80
succinylcholine 328
superior colliculus 243, 273
superior hypophyseal artery 45
superior orbital fissure 1, 2, 3
superior salivatory nucleus 6, 59
supraorbital artery 64
supraorbital nerve 5
supratrochlear artery 64
suxamethonium 215
sweat glands 301
sweating 323
Sylvian aqueduct syndrome 231,
    237
sympathetic nerves 58–9, 236, 315
sympathomimetics 232, 233
synaptic connections 274

T cells 115, 146, 149, 152, 190
    dependent antibody 151
    function 150
    tolerance 159–60
tamoxifen 194
tapeworm 121, 122
tarsal plates 9
tear
    biochemistry 198
    dynamics 197
    film 197
    production 196
    protein content 199
teeth 57
temporal arteries 77
temporal bone 71
tendinous ring 3
Tenon's capsule 34
Tensilon test 201
tetanus toxin 96
tetany 328
tetracaine 192
tetracyclines 127, 194
thioridazine 194, 195
thirst 302, 322
thrombocytopenia 132
thrombosis 165
    risk factors 164
thrombus formation 163
thymidine kinase 131

thymoxamine 234
thyroid arteries 77, 79
thyroid veins 79
thyroid gland 78–9
thyroidea ima artery 79
thyroglobulin 309–10
thyroglossal duct 78
thyroid hormones 309–11
thyroid stimulating hormone 309,
    311
tidal volume 307
timolol 185
topical medication 198
torsional movements 241
toxocariasis 122
Toxoplasma gondii 118, 123–4
trabecular meshwork 212, 213
trachoma 100, 127
transcortin 313
transplantation
    rejection 161–2
    tissue typing 160–1
    tolerance 159
    types 160
trichomonas 128
trichromats 291
trigeminal nerve 56, 57–8
trochlear nerve 3, 51, 52, 54
tropicamide 183
Troxler's phenomenon 245
tuberculosis 94, 144
tuberculous granuloma 145
tunica vasculosa lentis 24
tyrosine 257

ultraviolet radiation 90, 206, 211
uncal herniation 231
utricle 243
uveal tract 32
uveitis 98, 99, 193
uveoscleral outflow 184, 212

vagus nerve 59, 78
Valsalva manoeuvre 214
vanillylmandelic acid 316
varicellar zoster virus 107, 131
vasoconstriction 300, 301, 302
vasodilatation 300, 301, 302, 316
vena cava 299
ventilation perfusion ratios 308–9

vergence 243
Vernier acuity 279–80
version 243
vestibular-ocular reflexes 246
viruses 101
   airborne 109–112
   infection 103
   rapid diagnostic tests 104
   replication 102
   serology 104
   spread within host 104
   T cell activity 152
   transmission 103
vision
   blurred 238
   temporal properties 284–5
visual acuity and
     adaptation 277–89
   fovea-periphery 281–2
   newborn 283
   1 year old 283
   pupil size 281
visual adaptation *see* visual acuity
   and adaptation
visual cortex 46–7
   blood supply 48
   cell physiology 273
   visual field 275
visual deprivation 275–6
visual evoked potentials 269–271
visual field defects 46, 47
visual pathways 42–8, 272–6
   blood supply 45, 48
   lesions 45–6
vital capacity 307

vitamin A 194, 253–4, 310–11
   deficiency 98, 206
vitamin D 318
vitreous
   biochemistry 225
   collagen 226–7
   physical properties 224
   structure 225
vitrosin 225
vomiting 324–5
Von Michel's spur 25

Whitnall's tubercle 1
Windkessel effect 299
Wolfring glands 15, 197
wounds
   corneal 206
   healing 143–4, 314
   infections 98

X cells 273
xeroderma pigmentosum 175

Y cells 273
yeasts 118
yoked muscles 240

zidovudine 133
Ziehl-Neelsen stain 89
zonular fibres 22, 23, 30, 222
zoster viruses 104
zygomatic arch 71
zygomatic bone 1
zygomaticotemporal nerve 6